Stool Withholding:

What To Do When Your Child Won't Poop!

by Sophia J. Ferguson

First Edition (USA)
ISBN-10: 1505202140
ISBN-13: 978-1505202144

CONTENTS

INTRODUCTION

I was inspired to write this book after a grueling two year battle with my son's stool withholding. This is the book I needed then but couldn't find. If you and your child are going through this at the moment, I'm here to reassure you that you can, and *will*, overcome it.

Fortunately, you don't have to experience the prolonged struggle that my son and I endured. I will outline here everything you need to know about stool withholding and give you a straightforward approach to tackling it, with lots of tips and strategies to help you along the way.

Stool withholding is often triggered in a child by an episode of painful constipation. The child then becomes so terrified of experiencing this pain again that they hold on to their poop for days, even weeks, at a time. For some children this is a brief phase which passes quickly, while for others it becomes a long term issue requiring treatment.

This bewildering problem can sometimes feel like a form of daily torture, not just for the child but for the whole family. You may find yourself asking - how on earth can something as simple as having a poop be so extraordinarily difficult for my child?

Achieving a successful bowel movement with my son felt, at times, like coaching a woman through childbirth. When the event finally occurred there was huge relief and joy all round, only for the whole miserable experience to be repeated several days later. Unless you've experienced this nightmare with your own child, it's impossible to imagine just how distressing it can be.

Like many parents, I had never heard of stool withholding and thought my son was just severely constipated - a problem I could surely solve by myself. In my ignorance, I put off seeking medical help which delayed his recovery for much longer than necessary.

Stool withholding is still a widely misunderstood problem and some healthcare professionals are better informed about it than others. Finding the right advice can sometimes be challenging for parents. This was certainly my experience.

Without the right treatment, stool withholding can become an ingrained habit. If it's been going on for some time, it's unlikely to resolve all by itself and it's unlikely you'll magically figure out a solution on your own. Getting the right advice and support, as soon as possible, is therefore essential. Tackling it head on *now* will save you a lot of time and stress in the long term. I hope that by sharing my experience you can avoid some of the mistakes I made.

The good news is that the solution to your child's stool withholding is really quite straightforward. What you *will* need is the commitment to stick to a simple daily routine for many months or longer.

My son now uses the bathroom happily every day, without a trace of the fear and anxiety he experienced before. There were times when I thought we'd never achieve this outcome. Best of all, we now have a happy, relaxed and sociable child instead of the withdrawn and irritable one we lived with before. I'm confident this can be your outcome too.

While I have written this book primarily for parents, I hope it will also be useful to family doctors, pediatricians, nurses, teachers, social workers, nannies, foster parents, psychologists and anyone else who works with, or cares for, children. If awareness and understanding of this subject can be increased, perhaps many families can be spared the misery of this very distressing problem.

In writing this book, I have drawn not only on my own experiences with my son but on those of other parents too. Some of these parents were from my own circle of contacts and some I found through the many internet forums across the globe where parents discuss their childrearing issues.

The advice given here is also backed up by medical opinion and research. However, you should always seek the support of a healthcare professional in dealing with this issue and I would encourage you to do so as soon as possible.

There will be a lot of talk about "poop" and "pooping" to follow. I want this book to be as accessible to as many people as possible so have tried to avoid using technical terms. If you want to quickly extract the most useful advice, you'll find a summary of "Key Points" at the end of each chapter.

About Me

While I don't have the experience of a medical professional, I do have experience, as a parent, of dealing with a stool withholding child on a day-to-day basis. I also have a degree in Psychology, a Masters in Applied Social Research and a great interest in all things medical and psychological.

CHAPTER 1: What Is Stool Withholding?

Stool withholding is usually triggered in a child by anything that causes a bowel movement to be frightening, painful or distressing. The most common trigger is a bout of severe constipation.

If you've ever experienced severe constipation yourself, you'll know that passing a hard constipated stool can be extremely painful. If it's very severe, you may even receive a tear to your anus, known as an anal fissure, which leaves blood on the toilet paper after wiping. This tear can then reopen with subsequent stools, making the pain even more excruciating.

Experiencing this kind of pain can, understandably, cause some children to become terrified of having a bowel movement. This leads them to hold on for as long as they humanly can in an attempt to avoid this pain again. This is known as "stool withholding".

Soon, this holding-on becomes a knee-jerk reaction whenever the child feels an urge to go. In no time at all, a habit has formed which the child has little, or no, conscious control over.

The Vicious Circle

The longer a child holds on to their poop, the larger and more solid it becomes. As the stool sits in the intestine, water is drawn out of it into the body, making it harder and harder as each day goes by. The end result is a large, solid dry lump.

These large dried-out stools can be extremely painful to pass which causes the child to hold on for even longer. This leads to an even larger stool, which leads to more pain, which leads to more holding on, and so on and so forth. And so a nasty vicious circle begins which can be very hard to break.

Stretching of the Rectum

The longer your child holds on, the more their rectum (back passage) starts to stretch, much like a balloon, in order to hold the large lump of poop that is building up each day.

This stretching tends to interfere with the natural urges to go and it makes the muscles in the bowel less effective at pushing stools out. It also means there's now more room inside for a larger stool. So the longer your child holds on, the longer they are *able* to hold on.

At first, your child may only manage to hold on for a day or so, but as the months go by they'll be able to hold on for much longer periods. My son's record was about ten days. However, I've heard of children holding on for even longer than this.

We've all had times when we've had to hold on for a very short period of time. Even this can be extremely uncomfortable, but holding on for a week is unimaginable to most of us. In a bid to experience what my son was going through, I tried holding on myself but found it so unpleasant that I never managed more than a day.

Fortunately, your child's rectum should slowly shrink back to its original size once they start to have regular bowel movements. Over time, the natural urges to go should also return and the bowel should start to function normally again.

Fecal Impaction

Sometimes the stool that builds up in the child's intestine becomes so large and dry that it becomes almost impossible to pass. This is known as "fecal impaction". If the impaction is very severe, it can cause abdominal pain. The child may even vomit, although this is very rare and not something my son ever experienced.

If your child has been withholding for some time and has not been treated with any laxative medication, they will almost certainly have a large build-up of hard poop inside. Quite a high dose of laxative medication may be needed to flush the impaction out. We'll look at laxatives in detail in Chapter 5.

Soiling or Encopresis

Just to add to the misery, stool withholding often causes children to soil their underwear. This is usually known as "encopresis", or "retentive encopresis" to be precise to distinguish it from "non-retentive encopresis". The latter is a much less common type of soiling not usually associated with constipation or withholding.

Once a large impacted stool has formed in the intestine, softer poop tends to seep out around the hard lumps and into the child's underwear. Children have little, or no, control over this type of overflow soiling and are often quite unaware that it's happening. Scolding or punishing a child with this issue is, therefore, not appropriate or helpful.

Overflow soiling is usually soft or watery like diarrhea, but it's slightly different to the diarrhea we usually know. There's usually only a small amount, it often smells particularly foul, and it sometimes contains lumps. These lumps are small bits of the impaction which have fallen away.

Sometimes, however, the overflow soiling can be dry or grainy instead, rather than soft or watery. This was the type my son experienced in the form of dark-colored gritty skid marks in his underwear.

Not all children who stool withhold will experience encopresis. I was lucky that my son suffered only minor soiling. For some children, though, the soiling can be frequent and extremely messy. Leaving the home with a child who soils can be very stressful for parents and trips to the swimming pool become an impossibility.

Older children who soil are likely to experience great shame and embarrassment, and difficulty at school and in social situations. This is a thoroughly miserable problem for everyone involved.

Soiling is a classic sign of a child who is impacted and has been holding on for some time. Children who are impacted will also sometimes experience bed-wetting at night or leakage of urine during the day. This is because their rectum has become so enlarged that it starts to press against the bladder. Some children may also experience urinary tract infections if they develop a habit of holding on to their urine as well as their bowel movements.

With the right course of laxative medication, the hard impacted lump which is causing the soiling or wetting should shift quite quickly. This should resolve both of these issues, as long as the impaction can be prevented from reoccurring. A long term maintenance dose of laxatives is usually needed to avoid further impactions.

Soiling can, of course, also happen when a child is simply unable to hold on for any longer and has a full, or partial, bowel movement in their underwear. Sometimes this will happen during sleep. Once asleep, the child can't continue to hold on and so the stool passes by itself. This is obviously different to the type of overflow soiling which we've just talked about.

It's Not Constipation as we Know It

Even if your child is eating a high-fiber diet with plenty of fruit and vegetables, holding on to their poop for days at a time will still result in a hard constipated stool. So this is not constipation in the sense that we usually know it. The hard dried-out stools are not caused by diet but by your child holding on. And even if constipation was what triggered your child's withholding in the first place, it's very unlikely that changing their diet will stop them withholding, if the withholding has been going on for some time.

I spent the best part of a year filling my son up with fruit and vegetables in an attempt to cure what I thought at the time was severe constipation. However, these dietary improvements didn't make the slightest difference to his stool withholding.

I should stress, however, that avoiding constipation is a *very* important part of your child's long term recovery, particularly once they come off laxatives. A painful bowel movement could send them right back to square one. They need to be eating plenty of fruit, vegetables and other high-fiber foods and drinking enough fluids. Too much cow's milk can lead to constipation and we'll be discussing this in Chapter 3.

The Emotional Roller Coaster

The effect on your child's mood can be one of the most distressing aspects of stool withholding. As each day passes without a bowel movement, your child is likely to become more and more irritable and emotional. This is particularly so for younger children.

This distress usually comes in waves and then passes for a while, only to return in full force a few hours later. My son used to pace about rapidly and contort himself into strange positions during these very intense holding-on sessions. There would also be a great deal of screaming and crying which was harrowing to watch. My endless attempts to reassure him, and persuade him to go to the bathroom, made no difference whatsoever.

Going out in public was often very stressful when my son had been holding on for many days in a row. A wave of screaming and contorting could come at any moment and I had no idea how to explain this to other people.

Older children are usually better at controlling their emotions. However, if your child is a toddler, the emotional outbursts can be extreme. You may mistake these outbursts, as I did, for a bad case of the "terrible twos". In fact, it's the stool withholding which is making the terrible twos a hundred times *more* terrible than they really should be.

Stool withholding can also make your child lethargic. My son would often complain of tiredness and want to lie down rather than play or run about. He was also irritable much of the time, had a poor appetite and his sleep was disturbed. After a successful bowel movement, however, he would immediately come to life and for a day or so we would have a lively and happy child again.

Never Punish a Child for Stool Withholding

It's important to understand that your child is not holding onto their poop as an act of disobedience or willfulness. Nor is it likely to be an attention seeking tactic. They're usually doing it because they're genuinely terrified of having a bowel movement.

At times, you'll probably feel at your wits end with the whole issue. However, it's important to conceal your disappointment and frustration in front of your child and not to punish, scold or get angry with them. It always saddens me to hear of children being punished for their withholding and the soiling that often goes with it.

Stool withholding is an issue which requires great sensitivity and understanding on the part of parents. If you had a phobia of flying and your family punished and got angry with you and tried to force you onto a plane against your will, it would only create huge additional stress for you. You might well dig your heels in and refuse to cooperate at all.

When Does Stool Withholding Usually Start?

Stool withholding can begin at any age. It's even seen in babies of a few weeks of age. It seems to be most common in 2-4 year olds, but it can also start in school-age children. If left untreated it may continue well into the teens or beyond. Boys are a little more likely to stool withhold than girls.

How Common is Stool Withholding?

Stool withholding is a widespread problem and you'll have no trouble finding forums on the internet, across the world, full of anxious parents discussing this subject. You can rest assured that your child is not alone.

Quite how common it is we don't precisely know, because not enough research has been carried out. However, a study conducted in 1997 suggests that about one in eight children (12%) will go through a phase of stool withholding and about one in twenty (5%) will go on to develop a long term problem.[1] So, in a classroom of about twenty five school children, you'll probably find about three who have, or have had, an issue with stool withholding.

I remember being extremely reluctant and embarrassed to confide in friends and family about my son's withholding, thinking no one else would have heard of such a peculiar problem. Toileting habits are a bit of a taboo subject at the best of times. However, when I did finally open up, I was surprised at how many people either had experienced this issue in their own family, or knew of someone else who had. Stool withholding affects many families so there's no need to suffer in silence.

How Long Does Stool Withholding Take to Resolve?

The general guideline is that the length of time that your child has been stool withholding is usually the length of time that it takes for them to *stop* withholding, once the right course of treatment is started.[2]

In other words, if your child has been stool withholding for a year, it may take a further year from the day treatment begins for the problem to resolve completely. However, if you've already tried a course of treatment unsuccessfully, it's as if your child has not yet started treatment.[2]

If your child has been withholding for several years, please don't be disheartened by this news. This is just a rough guideline and you may be able to resolve things a little more quickly, as I did with my son. Children who start withholding as babies, however, sometimes take a bit longer to break the withholding habit than children who start at a later age.[2]

The good news is that once you find the right plan of action, which usually involves laxative medication, the extreme emotional roller coaster that your child may be going through now, could improve significantly within a matter of weeks. Once bowel movements start to become more frequent, the long and agonizing withholding sessions should soon be a thing of the past. You must then stick religiously to a simple daily routine for the foreseeable future. We'll be talking about what this routine entails in the chapters that follow.

CHAPTER 1: Key Points

- Stool withholding is usually triggered by anything which causes a bowel movement to be frightening, painful or distressing. A child starts holding on to their poop to avoid these feelings again. This causes stools to become large and hard, making them even more painful to pass, which causes the child to hold on even longer. A vicious circle then begins which can be very hard to break.

- Soiling, known as encopresis, is a common side effect of stool withholding. Soft poop seeps out around a hard impacted lump into the child's underwear. Occasionally, children also experience wetting if the impaction presses against their bladder. Shifting the impaction and preventing it from reoccurring with laxatives should resolve any soiling or wetting.

- Stool withholding is not an act of disobedience and nor is it an attention seeking tactic. Children usually withhold because they're genuinely terrified of having a bowel movement. They have little, or no, control over their withholding or the soiling and wetting that sometimes goes with it. Punishing a child for these issues is *not* appropriate or helpful.

- Stool withholding is not the same as constipation as we usually know it. Tackling the problem with diet, alone, is unlikely to help if your child has been withholding for many months. A long course of daily laxatives is usually the recommended way forward, along with the various strategies we'll be outlining.

- Avoiding constipation with high-fiber foods is still a *very* important part of your child's long term recovery and will help to prevent relapses once your child comes off medication.

- The length of time that your child has been stool withholding is usually the length of time it takes for them to *stop* withholding, once treatment is started. However, you may see a great improvement in your child's mood and behavior soon after starting laxatives.

CHAPTER 2: Is It *Really* Stool Withholding?

Stool withholding can be difficult to spot in children and is frequently mistaken for severe constipation, not only by parents but by healthcare professionals too. It can often take parents months, even years, to discover that their child is actually holding on to their poop.

Unfortunately, delaying treatment allows the withholding habit to become more deeply ingrained which can make it more difficult to resolve. It's therefore important to find out, as quickly as possible, if your child really is stool withholding so that the problem can be tackled in the appropriate way. Stool withholding is *not* the same as straightforward constipation and requires a different approach to treatment.

Children over the age of three will sometimes tell you themselves that they're holding on to their poop, but in younger children it can be much more difficult to diagnose. My son started stool withholding at about two and a half, but it took me a whole year to figure out what he was doing. Like many parents, I had never heard of stool withholding and assumed, as did my doctor, that we were simply dealing with severe constipation.

It was only after many hours of searching on the internet that I came across the term "stool withholding". Suddenly, my son's strange behavior and symptoms made sense. I remember the immense relief at realizing, finally, what the problem was and that I wasn't the only parent going through this ordeal.

Confusing Signs and Symptoms

The signs and symptoms associated with stool withholding can be extremely confusing for parents. When a child has overflow soiling it can look as though they have both diarrhea *and* constipation all at once. Also, a child who is in the middle of an intense holding-on session can sometimes look as though they're straining and parents naturally assume the child is constipated. This "straining", however, is not the child's attempts to force their poop *out*, but their desperate attempts to hold it *in*.

Confusion can again arise when a toddler refuses point-blank to poop on the potty. Parents often mistake this resistance for a toddler power struggle when, in fact, it's a withholding issue. Unless you've come across stool withholding before, you're unlikely to realize that all of these symptoms are due to your child holding on to their poop.

What are the Signs?

If you're not sure whether your child is stool withholding there are many telltale signs. Usually, a child will have some, or all, of the following symptoms:

- Infrequent bowel movements - less than three complete bowel movements per week with intervals of 2 to 7 days or more between each one;
- Huge resistance to sitting on the potty or toilet for pooping, with a great deal of crying and screaming in younger children;
- Your child may tell you that they're scared of pooping and may express intense fear at the prospect;
- Intermittent episodes of extreme crying, distress and irritability which escalates in the days leading up to a bowel movement;
- Your child may have sessions where they stand up on their tip-toes, pace about restlessly, strain, pull faces, fidget, clench their buttocks, contort their body, tense up, or grip onto furniture;
- Your child is restored to their happy, relaxed and lively self after a bowel movement;
- Leakage or soiling in the underwear of varying quantity and consistency. This is often soft or watery, may be particularly foul

smelling and may contain lumps. It can also sometimes be dry and gritty in consistency;

- Odd looking stools - these may be unusually large, wide in diameter, dark in color and of a clay-like consistency, and they may block the toilet;
- Leakage of urine during the day or bed-wetting at night due to an enlarged rectum pressing against the bladder;
- Urinary tract infections - these sometimes occur if a child also holds on to their urine in an attempt to stop bowel movements;
- Severe diaper rash in babies - the rash causes pain which makes the baby hold on;
- Young children may insist on having a diaper for pooping and will refuse to poop in the potty or toilet - this is a phase some children go through *before* the stool withholding habit begins;
- Children in diapers may go off to hide in a quiet corner of the room to have a bowel movement - again, this is a phase some children go through *before* the stool withholding habit begins;
- Tiredness and lack of energy - wanting to lie down and rest with little enthusiasm for physical activities or play;
- Reduced appetite - children sometimes learn that a meal triggers the urge for a bowel movement so will limit their food intake;
- A distended or bloated abdomen due to fecal impaction - a doctor may be able to feel the impaction in your child's abdomen;
- Anal fissures - small tears in the skin at the opening of the anus;
- Trapped gas and frequent passing of gas;
- Painful bowel movements;
- Abdominal pain or cramps;
- Disturbed sleep.

Children Who Partially Stool Withhold[3]

Just to confuse parents and doctors even further, occasionally children will *partially* stool withhold. In other words, they will still have regular, even daily, bowel movements but will hold on to a small amount of stool each time. This failure to completely empty the bowel eventually results in the child becoming impacted, which in turn may lead to soiling.

So, if your child has a soiling problem but *is* having regular bowel movements, they could still have a stool withholding issue and they may also be impacted.

What are the Signs in Babies?

Stool withholding can be particularly hard to spot in babies. Occasionally, babies who are stool withholding will look as if they're having a seizure or convulsion. It's not unheard of for parents to rush to the emergency department, suspecting epilepsy, only to discover that their child is stool withholding.[4] Stool withholding in babies is also occasionally mistaken for gastro-esophageal reflux.

Babies will sometimes behave in the following way during a withholding session:

- appear vacant, unresponsive or stare into space
- twitch or shake their arms and legs
- pull their legs up to their chest
- turn red or purple in the face
- stretch their back out
- roll their eyes
- clench their fists
- grimace and pull faces.

Severe diaper rash is sometimes a trigger for stool withholding in babies. The rash causes pain during a bowel movement and further pain during wiping. Some babies learn that holding on is a way to avoid this pain.

What About Older Children?

Stool withholding can also be difficult to spot in older school-age children. If your child is over seven or eight years of age, you may not know when, or how often, they go to the bathroom and they may be very good at hiding their withholding from the family.

Older children, however, are just as likely to experience soiling as younger children if the withholding has been going on for some time. If you spot any soiling in your child's underwear, this is a clear sign that they may be stool withholding.

A sensitive chat with your child may bear fruit. You can reassure them that it's not their fault and that this is a common problem which affects many children, for which there is a straightforward solution.

Don't Delay Seeking Help

It's important to determine as quickly as possible if your child is stool withholding. The checklist of symptoms in this chapter should help. If you have even the slightest suspicion, consult your family doctor or pediatrician straight away. A proper medical assessment will determine if your child really is withholding. Catching this issue early will lead to a speedier recovery.

CHAPTER 2: Key Points

- Stool withholding can be difficult to spot in children, particularly in babies and older school-age children. The symptoms can be confusing and both parents *and* healthcare professionals often mistake the signs for severe constipation. Stool withholding is *not* the same as straightforward constipation and requires a different approach to treatment.

- Sometimes a stool withholding child will look as though they're straining to push their poop *out* when, in fact, they're desperately trying to hold it *in*. And when a young child refuses to sit on the potty, parents often mistake this for a toddler power struggle when, in fact, it's a stool withholding issue.

- There are a whole range of signs and symptoms seen in children who stool withhold. These include infrequent bowel movements, soiling, large and wide clay-like stools, a distended abdomen, refusing to sit on the potty/toilet, and episodes of extreme emotional distress. (See pages 20-21 for a full list of symptoms).

- Occasionally, children will *partially* stool withhold. They may be having regular bowel movements but will hold on to a small amount of stool each time. Eventually, this can lead to an impaction which, in turn, can lead to soiling.

- Babies sometimes twitch, roll their eyes, pull faces and appear unresponsive during a withholding session. Parents have been known to mistake these movements for an epileptic seizure.

- It's important to seek medical help, as soon as possible, if you have even the slightest suspicion your child is stool withholding. The longer you delay tackling this problem, the more ingrained the habit is likely to become.

CHAPTER 3: Why Do Children Stool Withhold?

In this chapter, we'll look at why children usually start stool withholding. You'll find some important advice here if your child is at the toilet training stage or starting school or preschool.

What Usually Triggers Stool Withholding?

Stool withholding can begin for a variety of reasons. Occasionally, a traumatic or distressing incident can act as a trigger. I heard of one little boy whose dog was run over by a car just as he rushed into the house to have a bowel movement. He came to associate this upsetting event with using the bathroom and started holding on for fear of experiencing this distress again. I also heard of a little girl who started withholding after soiling herself in front of her classmates during a bout of stomach flu. The shame and humiliation she felt prompted her to start holding on.

The most common triggers for stool withholding, however, appear to be:

A) Painful constipation
B) Toilet training
C) Starting school or preschool

Sometimes more than one of these triggers will occur at the same time. In my son's case, all three coincided at once. We'll look at each of these now in turn.

A) PAINFUL CONSTIPATION

The most usual trigger for stool withholding is a very painful bout of constipation. This can prompt some children to start holding on in an attempt to avoid this terrible pain again.

I still remember my son's bloodcurdling screams, at the age of two and a half, as he struggled to pass a hard rock-like stool. After the event, I found traces of blood in his diaper. Although I didn't realize it at the time, this day marked the beginning of the stool withholding nightmare.

Cow's Milk and Constipation

With hindsight, I realize my son's severe constipation was almost certainly caused by too much cow's milk in his diet. At two and a half, he was still regularly demanding milk from a bottle and I'd had little success in breaking this habit. At this stage, he was still waking frequently in the night, and in my sleep-deprived state I gave in to his demands for milk much more than I should have. Had I been aware that too much cow's milk could cause constipation, I'd have weaned him from the bottle very swiftly indeed.

There are several reasons why cow's milk causes constipation. When a child fills up on milk they tend to be less hungry and less thirsty, so they'll reduce their intake of food and other fluids. This means less fiber and water in their diet which can result in constipation. Calcium and several of the proteins in cow's milk are also thought to contribute to constipation.

Cut Down on Dairy Products

It's important not to eliminate dairy products completely as they are a necessary part of your child's diet. Milk is an important source of Vitamin D and calcium. However, *too* much cow's milk or other dairy products, such as cheese or yogurt, can lead to constipation.

To give you a rough guideline, the recommended daily intake of milk or dairy products, per day, is as follows:[5,6]

| 1-8 year olds: | 2 servings |
| 9-18 year olds: | 3 servings |

One serving is equal to about 8½ fluid ounces of milk (250mls), 2oz of cheese (50g) or 8oz of yogurt (250g).

So, for example, a glass of milk, a 1oz slice of cheese (25g) and a 4oz serving of yogurt (125g) should be sufficient dairy intake, in one day, for a child between one and eight years of age.

Be aware that butter, margarine, cream, ice cream and chocolate all contain dairy products. If your child is having a lot of these foods, they may be having more dairy than you realize and these items should be reduced or cut out.

In my ignorance, I allowed my son to have a great deal more than the recommended two servings of dairy a day. I believe this is what caused the very severe episode of constipation which triggered his stool withholding.

Constipation in Babies

Breast milk is unlikely to cause constipation in babies. However, babies do sometimes become constipated during a period of weaning: either the introduction of solid food, or moving from breast milk to formula, or from formula to cow's milk. These changes can sometimes lead to constipation which can then trigger stool withholding.

Constipation and Milk Protein Intolerance

Occasionally, babies and young children can become constipated due to a milk-protein intolerance or allergy. While diarrhea is the *usual* symptom in children with a milk allergy, some children develop constipation instead.[7] (A milk allergy is not the same as lactose intolerance. Symptoms of lactose intolerance rarely occur in children before the age of about five).

There are several non-milk alternatives to formula and cow's milk on the market. You should, however, always consult a doctor before making any change to your child's milk.

What Else Causes Constipation?

Constipation is extremely common in young children. If you think constipation is what initially triggered your child's stool withholding, it helps to pinpoint what may have caused this constipation so that you can prevent it reoccurring.

We know that too much dairy or too little fiber in the diet often leads to constipation. However, there are various other causes which include:

- Dehydration
- Being ill with a fever
- Spending a lot of time in bed or lying down
- Lack of exercise
- A change of routine or diet, e.g. going on vacation
- Stressful life events
- Fussy or selective eating
- Certain medications
- Emotional stress
- Eating less

Some children do seem to be more prone to constipation than others. We know, for example, that children with cerebral palsy, Down syndrome and autism are more likely to experience constipation and are, therefore, more likely to stool withhold.

Very occasionally, chronic constipation can be a symptom of a more serious disorder such as Hirchsprung's disease, cystic fibrosis, hypothyroidism or celiac disease. These disorders are extremely rare. However, if your child has been battling with severe constipation for a long time, a thorough medical investigation is essential.

B) TOILET TRAINING

Toilet training is another common trigger for stool withholding. Moving from diaper to potty, or potty to toilet, can be very stressful for some children, particularly if training is rushed or pressured, or if it's started before a child feels ready.

Letting go of the poop into the gaping chasm of the potty or toilet can sometimes cause a child distress and they may resist this step by holding on. Even the sight of their poop can be frightening. If you've usually whisked your child's dirty diaper away out of sight, they may never have seen their own poop before. Let them have a good look and reassure them that it's not something to be afraid of.

Training my son for urine couldn't have been easier. However, pooping was a very different story and I believe I was guilty of rushing his toilet training *and* training him before he was ready.

Rushing Toilet Training in Time for Day Care or Preschool

Parents sometimes rush toilet training so that their child is trained before they start day care or preschool. My son started part-time day care at two and a half and I remember racing to get him out of diapers before his first day, pressuring him to complete toilet training in a couple of weeks, rather than several months.

However, this was not a deadline the day care center had imposed on me at all. In fact many, if not most, of the children there were still in diapers at two and a half. Day care staff *expect* to change diapers in young children - they're trained to do so and will usually help to toilet train your child.

So this was a deadline I had placed on my son quite needlessly. Unfortunately, I had absolutely no idea at this stage that stool withholding was a possible consequence of my rushed and pressured toilet training.

Why Did I Rush Toilet Training?

I think I rushed toilet training because I feared I'd be seen as an incompetent mother if my son was not trained by the age of two and a half. I'd had no success with his sleeping and fussy-eating and was desperate to prove to myself, and everyone else, that I could succeed in at least one area of motherhood.

Of course my anxieties were quite unnecessary. The average age for completing daytime toilet training is usually about 36 months.[8,9] In fact, around 40% of children aren't daytime toilet trained until they're *over* three years.[1] I could easily have delayed training for another six months, even longer, without appearing to be an "incompetent" mother.

However, it probably wasn't so much the age at which I started my son's training which contributed to his stool withholding, but rather the pressure I put on him to complete training in such a short period of time. He was also severely constipated at this stage *and* had the additional stress of starting day care. I believe all of these stresses combined together to create the perfect recipe for stool withholding.

Ignore Peer or Family Pressure to Toilet Train Your Child

The moral of the story is not to rush your child's toilet training or to be influenced by peer or family pressure to train your child by a particular age or deadline. If your child is resistant, it's best to leave training for several months and wait until they seem ready or show an interest. The more pressure you put on them, the more likely they are to resist.

Toilet training should take place over months rather than weeks. The key is to start a relaxed and gentle routine, without any pressure to perform, sitting your child on the potty once or twice a day at a set time with plenty of praise and rewards. Don't suddenly abandon the diaper, as I did, without several months of practice on the potty beforehand.

All children are different and some complete toilet training earlier and more easily than others. There's a huge variation, particularly across cultures, in the age at which children complete day-time training. This can range from about 22 months to 4½ years.[8] Children who stool withhold often train later than average, and boys often take a bit longer than girls, but they all get there in the end.

If you do feel under pressure from anyone to toilet train your child by a particular age, lend them this book and they will understand the very challenging issue you are dealing with.

Delay Toilet Training if Necessary

If your child is showing signs of stool withholding and you are about to start toilet training, or are in the early stages of training, research shows that delaying training and keeping your child in diapers, for the time being, often helps to resolve the withholding.[1] If this seems like a backward step, rest assured, it could save you and your child a *great* deal of time and distress in the long term.

It's vital to ensure that constipation and withholding have been resolved *before* you start toilet training. Your child may need laxative medication at this stage if their stools are hard and infrequent. A mild laxative such as lactulose may bring results. However, a stronger laxative may be needed if you suspect your child has been withholding for some time.

You should also ensure that your child is getting enough fruit, vegetables and other high-fiber foods in their diet and not too much dairy (see Chapter 6 for advice on diet).

Wait until your child has been having easy, regular and pain-free bowel movements, ideally once a day, for at least 2-3 months *before* you begin toilet training.

Will Poop in the Diaper but *Not* in the Potty

About one in four children will go through a phase of refusing to poop in the potty or toilet and will only poop in a diaper.[8,10] These are children who are *already* trained for urine and no longer in daytime diapers. This is a very common issue, sometimes known as "stool toileting refusal". (Some potty refusers may soil their underwear rather than request a diaper).

Many stool withholders appear to go through this potty refusing phase (about 80% in one study).[1] You may well have experienced this with your own child. Research shows that most potty refusers have been suffering with constipation *before* they start to refuse the potty.[8] In other words, constipation seems to be at the heart of the problem and is nearly always present well before any toileting problems begin.

Parents often mistake this potty resistance for a toddler power struggle. However, it's much more likely to be your child's way of dealing with the pain and discomfort of constipation. Getting angry or punishing a child who is refusing the potty is, therefore, not helpful and will only add to their misery.

This potty refusal is exactly what I experienced with my own son when I started toilet training. He would refuse with all his might to poop on the potty and would only perform with a diaper on. I went along with this regime for a while but with day care looming, to my great regret, I forced him to give up the diaper completely. That's when the stool withholding really set in.

Looking back, I can see that my son had probably been mildly constipated for many months before this potty refusal began - I just hadn't been aware of it. Severe constipation doesn't usually appear out of the blue but tends to develop gradually.

Let Potty Refusers Use a Diaper for Pooping

If your child is trained for urine and refuses to poop in the potty, but will poop happily in a diaper, the recommended way forward is to let them continue using a diaper just for pooping, for the time being. If you don't allow this they may start to stool withhold, if they haven't already started. The slight inconvenience of using a new diaper each time your child needs to go is nothing compared to the misery of stool withholding.

The next essential step is to tackle constipation if you suspect this is an issue. Pay close attention to your child's diet and their dairy and fluid intake. Again, a mild laxative such as lactulose may bring results at this stage. However, a stronger laxative may be needed if you think your child has been withholding for more than a few months.

Again, wait until your child has been having easy, regular and pain-free bowel movements, ideally once a day, for at least 2-3 months *before* you attempt to wean them from the diaper.

Weaning Your Child From the Diaper[3]

The best way to wean a potty-resistant child from the diaper is to take small and gradual steps. First, encourage them to go into the bathroom when they need a poop, while wearing a diaper. Once this has been mastered comfortably, encourage them to sit down on the potty or toilet while wearing a diaper.

Next, try cutting a small slit in a diaper and allow your child to wear this while they sit on the potty or toilet. Then, try cutting progressively larger holes over the course of several weeks. The slower you take this the more likely they are to succeed. Offering small rewards for each success can help this process along.

Some children dislike the sensation of their poop falling into the bowl of the toilet or potty, so placing some toilet paper into the bowl can help.

Why Will They Poop in a Diaper but *Not* in the Potty?

We don't exactly know why some children refuse the potty in favor of the diaper. As we've seen, most children who do this have a history of constipation. Perhaps pooping in a diaper is familiar and reassuring at a time when bowel movements are painful and frightening. Or, it could be that pooping in the standing-up position, with a diaper on, is less painful when constipated than sitting down on the potty.

My own hunch is that for some children refusing the potty may also be about a need for privacy. We know that hiding while pooping is very common in young children. As many as 70% of children who are still in diapers will go off to a private area, perhaps behind the sofa or a quiet corner of the room, in order to have a bowel movement.[9] When using the potty or toilet, however, they *can't* walk off and hide *and* there's usually an anxious parent hovering nearby who's pressuring them to perform.

Research shows that children who hide like this are, once again, frequently suffering with constipation.[9] I suspect the need for privacy becomes even more important for a child who is trying to deal with the pain and discomfort of constipation.

Hiding and the Need for Privacy

From the age of about twenty months, while still in diapers, my son used to hide whenever he needed to poop. He would disappear behind a chair in the corner of the room and signal for me to leave. He would not perform until he was certain I'd left the room and the door was firmly closed.

By the age of three, he'd learnt how to lock the bathroom door and I'd be refused entry. Pooping for him has always been, and still is, a very private matter indeed. This seems to be the case for quite a lot of children, particularly those that stool withhold.

Like most parents, I didn't give my son any privacy when he started toilet training. Instead, I tended to fuss around him nervously, urging him on and offering words of reassurance. I believe this lack of privacy was yet another factor which made him want to hold on.

Privacy while having a bowel movement is something most adults prefer too. I suspect it may just be a basic human instinct that's wired into many of us. There may even be evolutionary reasons for this which we won't go into here.

Giving your child privacy while they're pooping may help them to relax, let go and achieve the desired result. I believe, for some children, this is an important part of overcoming their withholding.

Warning Signs for Stool Withholding

For most parents reading this, it's too late to be talking about *preventing* stool withholding. However, I think it's important to highlight the two early warning signs for stool withholding that we've just mentioned:

1) refusing to use the potty for pooping and insisting on using a diaper instead; and/or
2) going off to hide in order to poop in the diaper.

If we can educate parents and healthcare professionals to keep an eye out for these two easy-to-spot signs, I believe many cases of stool withholding could be prevented. These two signs are also useful clues to help *confirm* a diagnosis of stool withholding.

Children who do one, or both, of these, as my son did, are much more likely to be constipated and more likely to start stool withholding, if they haven't already started. Not all stool withholders go through these two phases, but many do.

Constipation should be tackled immediately in these children with diet and, if necessary, with laxatives. In addition, they should have their toilet training put on hold, or be allowed to use a diaper just for pooping, until bowel movements have been easy and regular for at least 2-3 months. Giving them some privacy while they poop may also be very helpful.

C) STARTING SCHOOL OR PRESCHOOL

Sometimes children start to stool withhold when they begin school or preschool. They may feel uncomfortable using the bathroom there for bowel movements and start withholding to avoid going during school hours.

This is a surprisingly common issue. Research suggests that as many as 60% of school children will avoid using the school bathroom for bowel movements.[11,12] This may be about the need for privacy which we've just talked about. School bathrooms usually offer little privacy *and* they're often rather unpleasant, dirty and uncomfortable places too.

Develop an Evening "Toilet Sit" to Avoid School Hours

I was lucky to have resolved my son's stool withholding just before the start of school. However, he refused to use the school bathroom for well over a year after starting school, and still isn't keen on using it to this day, even for urine.

One of the most useful bits of advice I can give to any parent of a stool withholding child who is already toilet trained is to train them to poop in the evening. This greatly reduces the need to go during the day when they're at school or preschool. I believe this played a key role in my son's recovery.

You could of course opt for a morning "toilet sit". This might suit better if you're an early riser and can ensure your child won't be rushed or pressured. Whether you choose morning *or* evening, the most important thing is to set a routine and stick to it at the *same* time *every* day. It may take a while to train your child to go at this set time but the more you practice, the more the habit will take hold.

My son's evening toilet sit, which he continues with today, means that the need for a bowel movement during school hours rarely, if ever, arises. This greatly reduces the risk of the withholding habit being triggered again while at school. It also means I can relax knowing that he won't be going through the misery of holding on at school.

The daily toilet sit is such an important part of your child's recovery that we'll be talking about it in more detail in Chapter 6.

Avoiding the School Bathroom

The evening (or morning) toilet sit does, of course, avoid confronting your child's dislike of the school bathroom. If you want to tackle this, it can help to gently encourage your child to practice using bathrooms outside the home.

If your child is just starting school or preschool, it's also a very good idea to take them to the bathroom there a few times yourself to ease their anxieties. I wish I had done this with my son. Offering rewards can be helpful if your child is very resistant to trying this.

Children usually grow out of this early resistance to the school bathroom. I remember going through a brief phase of this myself. My son still dislikes the school bathroom but he will now use it if he really needs to.

CHAPTER 3: Key Points

- The most common triggers for stool withholding are constipation, toilet training and starting school or preschool.

- Drinking too much cow's milk can lead to constipation. Milk and other dairy products should not be eliminated but kept to within the recommended daily amount (see page 27).

- Toilet training can trigger stool withholding if it's rushed or pressured, or started before a child feels ready. Training should take place over months rather than weeks. Try to ignore peer or family pressure to toilet train your child by a particular age.

- Toilet training should be put on hold if your child is showing signs of stool withholding or constipation. Avoid training until both of these issues have been resolved and your child has had 2-3 months of easy, regular and pain-free bowel movements.

- If your child will poop in a diaper but not in the potty or toilet, allow them to continue using a diaper for pooping. Again, wait until they've had at least 2-3 months of easy, regular and pain-free bowel movements before slowly weaning them from the diaper.

- Children who go off to hide before pooping in the diaper, and those who refuse the potty for pooping in favor of the diaper, are much more likely to be constipated *and* more likely to develop a stool withholding problem (if they haven't already). Tackling constipation early in these children could prevent many from developing a withholding issue.

- Like adults, many children have a need for privacy while pooping. Giving your child privacy may help them to relax and let go, which is an important part of recovery for some children.

- Children sometimes start withholding while at school/preschool because they dislike using the bathroom there. A scheduled daily "toilet sit" for pooping in the evening, or morning if preferred, greatly reduces the need to go during school hours. If your child is just starting school/preschool, it's a good idea to take them to the bathroom there a few times to ease their anxieties.

CHAPTER 4: Parents' Common Concerns

The purpose of this chapter is to ease any concerns you may have about your child's stool withholding. If your child has been withholding for some time, the problem has probably become a source of great anxiety, dominating your family's thoughts and conversation on a daily basis.

I wasted a great deal of time worrying needlessly about the whole issue. Learning to relax and feel optimistic will help your child to relax and feel optimistic too. I believe this is an important part of your child's recovery.

It's Not Your Fault!

Mothers are often quick to blame themselves when their children experience a problem. I'm certainly guilty of this myself. However, your child's stool withholding is definitely not your fault, and nor is it in any way a reflection of your parenting style or abilities.

Most parents have never heard of stool withholding, so unless you happen to have been an expert on the subject before you experienced it with your own child, there's simply no way you could have anticipated the problem, or prevented it from arising. Remarkably, even after four years of studying psychology at university, I never encountered the subject of stool withholding.

Could There be Something Psychologically Wrong?

One of my biggest anxieties was that my son's stool withholding was a symptom of an underlying psychological or emotional problem. I worried that perhaps he was withholding because he was unhappy or anxious for some reason. I also worried about his extreme emotional outbursts which I wasn't seeing in any of my friends' children. Let me quickly reassure you that it's very unlikely that there's anything psychologically or emotionally wrong with your child.

A reassuring study conducted in 1997, compared the behavior of children who refused to poop on the potty with the behavior of children without this toileting difficulty.[13] No differences were found in the behavior of the two groups of children and the toilet refusers were no more likely to have behavioral problems than the non-toilet refusers. Similarly, research shows that children with retentive encopresis usually have no underlying behavioral or psychological issues.[14]

We also know that counselling or psychotherapy has little or no benefit when it comes to stool withholding.[15] In other words, getting your child to talk to a counselor or psychologist about their life and how they feel, won't stop them stool withholding. This indicates that stool withholding is not caused by any underlying emotional or psychological problem.

Most of your child's difficult behavior will be due to the extreme discomfort of holding on to their poop for long periods of time. Once the stool withholding has resolved, their mood and behavior will almost certainly transform.

Holding on for many days at a time will make even the most angelic child a nightmare to live with. And, if it's coinciding with the "terrible twos" when children are often extremely troublesome anyway, you may feel like you've produced the child from hell.

In the unlikely event that any extreme behavior continues *after* the stool withholding has been resolved then you should, of course, seek appropriate advice and support for this.

It's a Learned Behavior Not a Psychological Problem

I believe stool withholding is a child's logical reaction to intense pain or fear. If you associate anything with pain or fear, you naturally want to avoid it at all costs.

Some children quickly learn that they can avoid the pain and fear of pooping if they squeeze tight whenever they feel an urge to go. Soon, this squeezing tight develops into a reflex which happens automatically in response to the slightest urge to poop - what psychologists call a "conditioned reflex".[3] The longer the habit goes on, the more automatic and reflexive it becomes. The child can no longer control it and may not even be aware that they're doing it. Like any habit, it takes time and a great deal of repetition to *unlearn* the old habit of squeezing tight and to *relearn* the new habit of relaxing and letting go.

Some of us are a little more sensitive to, and fearful of, pain than others. My son and I seem to fall into this category, but it doesn't mean that there's anything psychologically wrong with us. However, I suspect it does mean that some children are a bit more prone to stool withholding than others.

Is Stool Withholding Dangerous?

Stool withholding is not dangerous or life threatening. Your child's intestine will never burst or rupture, even after holding on for long periods. The rectum *is* likely to become enlarged and less efficient at pushing stools out, but it should gradually shrink back to its natural size and return to normal functioning once your child fully recovers. It's unlikely any permanent damage will result.

However, as we've already stressed, it's still essential to seek medical help for your child's withholding as quickly as possible. The longer it goes on, the more your child's rectum will stretch and the more ingrained the withholding habit will become.

Could There be a Serious Physical Problem?

Parents often worry that there might be an underlying physical problem such as a blockage in the bowel or a hernia which is causing their child's terrible discomfort and distress. Again, let me reassure you that this is very unlikely.

Your family doctor or pediatrician should look at all of your child's symptoms carefully to rule out anything serious and will probably have a good feel of your child's abdomen. In the unlikely event that they do suspect a physical problem, they may refer your child for an x-ray or other investigation.

As Dr Anthony Cohn points out in his excellent book "Constipation, Withholding and Your Child", parents tend to worry more about a physical problem the *longer* the stool withholding has been going on.[2] However, "serious stuff gets worse over time" he says, so the longer your child has been withholding the *less* likely it is to be anything serious.

In other words, if your child had a twist or a blockage in their bowel or a trapped hernia you would know about it pretty quickly - they would be in severe pain and possibly vomiting. And bowel cancer is so rare in children that most doctors never encounter a single case during their careers.[2]

However, some symptoms should be taken seriously. If your child is experiencing weight loss, recurrent fevers, frequent chest infections or has blood in their stools, this may point to an underlying physical problem and a trip to the doctor should be your first priority.

Autism and Stool Withholding

After many hours of searching on the internet, I discovered that stool withholding is more common in children with autism and those on the autism spectrum. I immediately started worrying that my son might be autistic. I could tell he wasn't severely autistic but, for a while, I managed to convince myself he was on the very mild end of the spectrum (he isn't).

The reason stool withholding is more common in children on the autism spectrum, is because they're much more likely to suffer with constipation than non-autistic children.[16] Autistic children are therefore more likely to withhold because constipation is the most common trigger for stool withholding. Stool withholding is a symptom of constipation *rather* than a symptom of autism.

In fact, autistic children are much more likely to suffer with a whole range of digestive issues, including constipation, diarrhea and irritable bowel conditions. So, rest assured, there is no reason whatsoever to conclude that your child is autistic just because they're stool withholding. Constipation is also more common in children with Down syndrome and cerebral palsy, so stool withholding is seen more often in these children too.

If your child *is* on the autism spectrum, or has any other developmental issues, then treating stool withholding is essentially the same as it is for any child. You may well have other toilet training hurdles to overcome, for which I would recommend these books:

- *"Toilet Training for Individuals with Autism or Other Developmental Issues"* by Maria Wheeler;

- *"Ready, Set, Potty!: Toilet Training for Children with Autism and Other Developmental Disorders"* by Brenda Batts.

Your Child *Will* Overcome This

You may well have had times when you've felt utterly hopeless about your child's situation and feared that things will never get better. I felt this way myself on many occasions. I am certain, however, that if you carefully follow the advice in this book and seek the support of a healthcare professional who understands this issue, your child will conquer this. Adopting a relaxed and optimistic outlook along the way will also greatly assist you and your child.

CHAPTER 4: Key Points

- Your child's stool withholding is not your fault and has nothing to do with your parenting style or abilities.

- It's very unlikely that your child's withholding or encopresis is due to any underlying psychological or emotional issue. Stool withholding is usually a child's logical reaction to pain, fear or distress experienced during a bowel movement. Your child's mood and behavior should improve significantly once appropriate treatment is started.

- It's also very unlikely that your child has a physical issue such as a blockage or hernia. A serious issue would present very quickly as a medical emergency. However, it's still important that your child has a thorough medical assessment.

- Stool withholding is not dangerous and is unlikely to cause your child any permanent physical damage. It *can* cause the rectum to become temporarily enlarged and to become less efficient at pushing stools out, but this should gradually return to normal once bowel movements become frequent again.

- Children on the autism spectrum are much more likely to suffer with constipation. This means that stool withholding is seen more often in autistic children. However, stool withholding is a symptom of constipation and *not* of autism. Just because your child is stool withholding does not mean they are on the autism spectrum.

- Learning to relax and feel optimistic about your child's stool withholding will help your child to relax and feel optimistic too. This is an important part of helping your child recover.

CHAPTER 5: Laxative Medication

You can tell your child a thousand times over that they don't need to be scared of pooping, but it won't stop them holding on. They actually have to experience easy, pain-free bowel movements for themselves, *many* times over, and that's where laxatives help.

The word "laxative" used to refer to stimulant varieties, such as Senna, but now the term usually covers any medication which helps a bowel movement along its way. This is the definition we'll be using here.

Your child should, of course, only take laxatives under the close guidance and supervision of a healthcare professional.

Why Use Laxatives?

With the right dose, laxatives make it extremely difficult for your child to continue to hold on and they make bowel movements soft, regular and painless. This helps to break the nasty vicious circle of pain and fear.

Laxatives also help to flush out any hard impacted lumps. This allows the rectum to shrink back down to its regular size and the normal functioning of the bowel to return. With each pain-free bowel movement, your child slowly learns that pooping is no longer frightening or painful and, over time, they should start to relax and let go.

Does Your Child *Really* Need Laxatives?

If your child has been stool withholding for many months, or years, then a long course of laxative medication is usually the recommended way forward.[17] This may mean taking laxatives for *at least* six months or more, and often at quite a high initial dose. It's unlikely your child will simply "grow out" of their withholding if this has been going on for some time.

However, if your child has been withholding for *less* than a few months, you may achieve success with the strategies described in Chapter 6, along with a mild laxative such as lactulose. If this doesn't bring results quite quickly, it's important not to battle on needlessly for months - a stronger laxative may be needed. Remember, you must act quickly. The longer you delay tackling this head-on, the longer it can take to resolve.

Are Laxatives Safe?

The laxatives we'll be talking about are all safe to use with children, even at slightly higher doses and for longer periods than recommended on the product label. Parents should rest assured that the safety profile of laxatives today is extremely good and research backs this up.[18,19,20]

Parents often worry that their child will become dependent on laxatives for a bowel movement or that the gut will become "lazy". However, there appears to be no convincing evidence for this.[20]

There are, of course, guidelines on the appropriate doses for different laxatives and the length of time that they should be used for, which we'll come to in a moment.

Parents' Fears About Laxatives

Fears about the safety of laxatives often lead parents to stop their child's medication too soon, to give it on-and-off, to skip doses, to taper it off too quickly, or to give a dose that's simply too low to have any effect. Unfortunately, the end result is usually a child who relapses again and again over a period of years which draws the agony out for much longer than necessary. This is an extremely common trap which many parents, unintentionally, fall into.

Giving the medication to your child consistently every day, without fail, at the recommended dose, is the fastest route to recovery. In fact, over the long term, your child may end up taking *less* medication, in total, with this approach than if you adopt a stop-start approach over many years. Giving a dose sporadically, or that's too low, is often as good as doing nothing at all and simply wastes precious time.

I, too, was anxious about giving my son a high dose of laxative each day for many months. However, I was so desperate for a solution that I overcame my resistance and knuckled down to the job. My only regret is not starting it sooner. I suspect if I hadn't taken this route my son would still be struggling with this problem today.

Enemas & Suppositories

Enemas and suppositories used to be used routinely with children. However, most children, especially stool withholders, are very sensitive and private in relation to their bottoms, so intruding into that area can be extremely distressing. I believe suppositories and enemas should be avoided and used only as a last resort if your child is severely impacted and has had no success with oral laxatives. Oral laxatives are just as effective and much safer and less unpleasant for your child.

Which Laxatives are Most Effective for Stool Withholding?

There's a bewildering array of laxatives now available on prescription and over the counter. To keep things simple, I'll mention just a few of the most popular and effective ones for stool withholding.

Different laxatives work in slightly different ways but, with the right dose, they *all* have the same end-result of making it very difficult for your child to hold on, and this is the objective. One laxative, in particular, is extremely safe and effective when it comes to stool withholding so we'll look at this first.

Polyethylene Glycol 3350 (PEG): MiraLAX

Polyethylene Glycol 3350, or "PEG" for short, is one of the safest and most effective laxative medications for stool withholding. It usually goes under the brand name "MiraLAX" in the United States and "RestoraLAX" or "Lax-A-Day" in Canada. Many children across the world have achieved success with PEG and it certainly worked miracles with my son.

PEG is a powerful osmotic laxative known as a macrogol which holds onto water that is already in the bowel, making stools soft and lubricated. It is very safe to use with children and a number of studies back this up.[21,22] PEG is now usually recommended as a first-line medication for stool withholding and constipation in children.[17,23]

Reassuringly, PEG is expelled from the body once it has served its purpose and is virtually unabsorbed into the bloodstream. This makes it very safe for your child. It's also less likely to dehydrate the body than some other laxatives because it retains water that's already in the bowel, rather than drawing water out of the body.

Is it Safe to Take PEG for Long Periods?

Parents often worry about keeping their child on PEG for long periods of time. On the MiraLAX product label it states: "use no more than 7 days" which often causes parents great anxiety.

Several reassuring studies have shown that PEG is very safe for long term use in children.[24,25] In one study, children who had been taking PEG for up to two and a half years were monitored carefully, and detailed blood tests carried out while they were on the medication.[24] All blood tests came back normal.

I know of many children who have been on PEG continuously for several years without any adverse effects. Clearly, no parent wants their child to be on medication for a long time and hopefully your child won't have to be. However, the safety profile of PEG is very good and long term use, where necessary, is perfectly acceptable under medical supervision.

Does PEG Have Side Effects?

My son took PEG for six months, in total, and experienced no adverse side effects whatsoever. Many children take it for much longer than this without problems and usually experience few, if any, side effects.

Possible side effects include nausea, bloating, cramping and gas. If these do occur, they're often temporary and will wear off as your child adjusts to the medicine. Obviously, the medication should be stopped straight away if side-effects are causing a lot of distress - there are plenty of alternative laxatives available.

Can Babies Take PEG?

PEG is usually recommended for children *over* two years of age. However, doctors do prescribe it for babies, only in very small doses. Research shows that at low doses it can be used safely and effectively with babies from one month of age, under medical supervision.[26,27]

How Long Does PEG Take to Work?

PEG usually takes 1-3 days to trigger a bowel movement, but it may take longer if your child is a long term withholder, or very impacted. If little, or no, effect is seen after five days, then a higher dose is probably needed.

How to Take PEG

PEG comes in the form of a powder which needs to be dissolved in liquid. The powder can be mixed up in advance and stored for 24 hours in the fridge. PEG need not be taken with meals.

MiraLAX bottles come with a 17g dose measuring cap, as do RestoraLAX and Lax-A-Day bottles. Each capful, filled to the line, should be dissolved in about 4 to 8 ounces of fluid.

One 17g cap contains roughly 5 level teaspoons of powder. Using a teaspoon rather than the supplied measuring cap allows you to give a more precise dose. The type of measuring teaspoon used for cooking is recommended, rather than a household teaspoon.[3]

Strategies to Help Your Child Take PEG

I was lucky that my son drank his PEG, without complaint, dissolved in fresh orange juice. Most children have no problem taking PEG. However, some dislike the taste and this is where you need to be a little creative. The following strategies may help:

1. Dilute PEG with more fluid to disguise the taste. I dissolved my son's PEG in almost twice the recommended amount of fluid.

2. Let your child sip their PEG over the course of the day. This helps if your child objects to the volume of liquid that needs drinking, especially during the disimpaction stage.

3. I recommend the type of cup with a lid and a built-in straw. A straw can make drinking easier for children and the lid allows the mixture to be shaken up vigorously so that the powder is completely dissolved. If your child finds a gritty sludge at the bottom it can put them off drinking it, so it's important to mix it thoroughly.

4. It's well worth experimenting with different types and flavors of drink. Some parents achieve success with lemonade, cranberry juice, milk, flavored milk, smoothies or apple juice. Usually, the stronger the flavor the better. You can also mix PEG into drinking chocolate (use hot rather than boiling milk).

5. Dissolved PEG is usually more palatable served cold from the fridge, rather than at room temperature - adding ice cubes can also help.

6. Some parents achieve success with younger children by feeding them dissolved PEG with a syringe. You can also add it to a baby's bottle as long as it's completely dissolved first.

7. You can even add PEG to food, as long as the powder is dissolved first *before* adding. PEG dissolved in milk mixes well with oatmeal, breakfast cereals, and savory foods like mashed

potato and scrambled eggs. I've even heard of parents disguising PEG in jello and popsicles.

8. If you can, try to avoid telling your child you've put medicine in their food or drink - the thought of it can put them off.

What's the Right Dose of PEG?

There is no single dose of PEG that will suit all children. Every child is different and you will need to experiment to find the best dose for your child. A doctor should be able to advise you on the most appropriate dose. The doses of PEG suggested in this chapter are intended as a guide only and are based on those recommended by the National Institute for Health and Care Excellence (NICE).[17]

We're treating stool withholding, *rather* than straightforward constipation, so a higher dose than recommended on the label is usually needed. This can make your child's poops rather runny. However, this is usually a necessary step in the early stages of treatment, particularly for long term withholders, to make it as difficult as possible for them to hold on.

Shifting an Impaction with PEG

The first and most important step is to clear out any impaction or hard build-up of poop from your child's bowel. This is known as "disimpaction" and is an *essential* step in your child's treatment. If soiling is an issue, this should either stop straight away, or reduce in frequency, once the impaction is cleared. Soiling usually resolves completely once the rectum has returned to its normal size and functioning. This may take some time to achieve for longer term withholders.

If an impacted child is put straight onto a maintenance dose of laxative *without* the impaction being cleared first, progress will be extremely slow, if not non-existent. Signs of impaction include less than three complete bowel movements per week, soiling and a distended abdomen. A doctor may be able to feel the impaction in your child's abdomen. Children who are *not* impacted can move straight on to the maintenance dose of PEG.

Clearing an impaction usually takes about 3-7 days.[22] You will know that the clear-out is complete when no more hard lumps are visible and stools are of a liquid consistency. As soon as your child reaches this stage, they can drop straight down to the maintenance dose.

Typical disimpaction doses for MiraLAX are given opposite. The dose can be spread through the day rather than given all at once. Exactly the same doses apply for RestoraLAX and Lax-A-Day.

If your child is *under* two years, a doctor will advise on the most appropriate disimpaction dose.

MiraLAX Disimpaction Dose for 2-5 year olds:

	Level Teaspoons of MiraLAX*
Day 1	4 tsps
Day 2	8 tsps
Day 3	8 tsps
Day 4	12 tsps
Day 5	12 tsps
Day 6	16 tsps
Day 7	16 tsps

Continue until clear-out is complete. Move on to maintenance dose as soon as all hard lumps have disappeared.

MiraLAX Disimpaction Dose for 6-12 year olds:

	Level Teaspoons of MiraLAX*
Day 1	8 tsps
Day 2	12 tsps
Day 3	16 tsps
Day 4	20 tsps
Day 5	24 tsps
Day 6	24 tsps
Day 7	24 tsps

Continue until clear-out is complete. Move on to maintenance dose as soon as all hard lumps have disappeared.

* One 17g cap of MiraLAX (or RestoraLAX or Lax-A-Day) filled to the line, is equivalent to 5 level teaspoons of powder. Using a teaspoon (the type used for cooking) allows for more precise dosing.[3]

PEG Maintenance Dose

Once any impaction has been cleared, your child can move straight on to a maintenance dose of PEG. Again, the doses given below are for guidance purposes only. You will need to adjust the dose according to your child's response.

Doses can be divided into a morning and evening dose, or spread throughout the day, rather than given all at once. If your child is *under* two years, a doctor will advise you on the most appropriate maintenance dose.

Typical maintenance doses of MiraLAX are as follows (the same doses apply for RestoraLAX and Lax-A-Day):

2-5 years: Start with 2 level teaspoons of MiraLAX per day and increase by 2 teaspoons, every other day, to a maximum of 8 teaspoons per day, according to your child's response.

6-12 years: Start with 4 level teaspoons of MiraLAX per day and increase by 2 teaspoons, every other day, to a maximum of 8 teaspoons per day, according to your child's response.

It may take a few weeks of experimenting to find the right maintenance dose. The aim is to increase the number of bowel movements your child is having each week.

At least five complete bowel movements per week is a good target to aim for, initially, for children over three (or once a day for children *under* three). In the long term, we're aiming for about one daily bowel movement for all children.

Will PEG Cause Accidents?

As with any laxative, too much will turn your child's poop to liquid, and too little will have no effect at all. We want poops to be quite runny at first, to break the vicious cycle of pain and fear, but we don't want explosive accidents.

To my surprise, my son never experienced an accident while on PEG, even during the disimpaction phase. Long term withholders often develop an extraordinary ability to hold on. However, some children do have accidents, particularly during disimpaction.

You may want to use diapers or training pants with your child, just in case, in the early stages. Ideally, it's best to start the medication at a weekend, or during a holiday period, so that you can be at home to deal with any mishaps.

If necessary, take your child out of school or preschool for a few days while they adjust to the medication. Teachers should be made aware that this is a serious issue that needs tackling as quickly as possible. It can be very upsetting for a child to have accidents at school and teachers won't enjoy it either.

My Son's Experience on MiraLAX

My son took MiraLAX for a total of six months, starting at the age of three and a half. After clearing his impaction, we settled on a maintenance dose of 8 level teaspoons of MiraLAX, per day, for the first two months – four teaspoons dissolved in a large beaker of fresh orange in the morning, and the same again in the evening.

Eight teaspoons per day reduced his poops to a liquid consistency. I believe this high initial dose was an essential part of breaking the withholding vicious circle. In the third month we reduced the dose to six teaspoons per day to make things a little less runny.

My son's dosage, over six months, looked roughly as follows:

	Level Teaspoons of MiraLAX per day
Month 1:	8 tsps*
Month 2:	8 tsps
Month 3:	6 tsps
Month 4:	4 tsps
Month 5:	4 tsps
Month 6:	2 tsps
Slowly tapering off dose completely in Month 6	

* Started with 2 teaspoons of MiraLAX and increased by 2 teaspoons every other day to 8 teaspoons.

This is what worked for my son at the age of 3½ to 4 years after a whole year of withholding. Your own child may need an entirely different dose over a longer or shorter period depending on their age, weight and the length of time they've been withholding.

During this six month period on MiraLAX, my son's bowel movements increased from about one per week to five per week. All of his distress and resistance slowly disappeared during this time until eventually he was going to the bathroom happily and willingly most nights before bed.

I tried several times to stop the medication during the first three months, thinking we'd resolved the problem, but he immediately relapsed. He was clearly still trying his hardest to hold on at this stage.

After six months, he was no longer taking any medication and he continued to have about five soft, easy bowel movements per week, without any distress. I was delighted with this result and accepted that perhaps he wasn't going to be a once-a-day child. However, slowly over the next four months, *without* any medication, he went from five bowel movements per week to one every single day. I suspect this final improvement was due to his rectum shrinking back to its regular size and the functioning of his bowel returning to normal.

It, therefore, took a total of ten months, from the day my son started daily MiraLAX, before I really felt we had conquered the problem. However, I continued to stay vigilant for a couple of years after that, prompting him to go before bedtime each evening and keeping an eye out for constipation.

Not every child's road to recovery will be as straightforward as this. Some will take longer and some will resist the process much more than others. However, it does show the benefit of starting your child on a high maintenance dose of PEG, particularly if they've been withholding for some time. It always amazed me that even on eight teaspoons of MiraLAX per day, my son could still hold on for several days at a time.

Other Laxatives Suitable for Stool Withholding

PEG clearly comes out on top when it comes to treating stool withholding. However, if for any reason your child doesn't succeed with PEG, it's important to find an alternative quickly rather than waste weeks or months struggling unsuccessfully. There are many other laxatives available and we'll look at a few of these next.

1. Stimulant Laxatives

Stimulant laxatives work by making the muscles in the gut contract more often so that stools are pushed along with more force. Parents often worry that stimulant laxatives will harm their child. However, research shows that, used appropriately, this group of laxatives is very safe.[18,19]

Stimulant laxatives tend to produce a powerful urge for a bowel movement. Long term stool withholders often lose awareness of the urge to go, so stimulants can help to remind them of this important sensation.

Abdominal cramps are a common and unpleasant side effect of

stimulant laxatives so it's very important to start with a low dose and see how your child reacts *before* increasing the dose. If they experience too much discomfort, stop the medication straight away.

Stimulant laxatives are suitable for short term use only and should never be taken continuously for more than 12 months.

Combining a Stimulant Laxative With Another Variety

Stimulant laxatives can be taken on their own but they often work well when combined with another type of laxative. For example, some children struggle to drink the volume of liquid that needs to be taken with PEG, particularly during disimpaction. In this instance, a stimulant laxative can be taken *alongside* PEG. This means you can *reduce* the dose of PEG and add one of the stimulant laxatives listed next.

Stimulant laxatives can also be combined effectively with a stool softener or lubricant laxative (we'll look at these varieties in a moment). A doctor should be able to advise you on the appropriate doses of each laxative if you want to combine two different types.

Stimulant laxatives sometimes come in the form of a liquid or syrup. Usually, only one small daily dose is required which makes them much easier for children to take than PEG.

The following stimulant laxatives are safe to use either on their own, or in combination with another laxative:

- **Senna**

  Senna is a strong stimulant laxative which is usually taken once a day. For children, it often comes as a sweet-tasting liquid or syrup and takes about 6-12 hours to have an effect. A common brand name in the United States is "Fletcher's Laxative". Due to its strength, Senna is not usually recommended for children under two years.

- **Bisacodyl**

  Bisacodyl is a *very* strong stimulant laxative. It is not recommended for children under 4 years. It is usually taken in tablet form, once a day, and takes about 6-12 hours to have an effect. Tablets must not be broken, crushed or chewed.

2. **Stool Softeners and Lubricant Laxatives**

Stool softeners and lubricant laxatives soften or lubricate stools so that they pass along the gut more easily. These types of laxative can be taken on their own but also work well when combined with one of the stimulant laxatives we've just mentioned. Two common varieties include:

- **Docusate Sodium**

  Docusate Sodium is a "stool softener" which allows water to penetrate hard stools, making them softer and easier to pass. It can be combined with a stimulant laxative and can also be taken alongside PEG. However, it should never be taken with mineral oil.

  Docusate Sodium usually comes as a liquid which needs to be taken three times a day, diluted in a glass of water, juice or milk. It can take about 1-3 days to have an effect. It's not usually recommended for children under 6 months.

- **Mineral Oil**

  Mineral oil is a "lubricant laxative". It coats stools with a waterproof film which helps them to slide out more easily. This is an old fashioned, over-the-counter, remedy which is still popular in the United States for constipation.

  Mineral oil has few side effects and can be used safely for long periods. It usually takes 6-10 hours to have an effect. Mineral oil should *never* to be taken with docusate sodium. However, it can be combined safely with a stimulant laxative.

Inhaling mineral oil *can* cause damage to the lungs. Although the risk of inhalation is very small, mineral oil should only be given when a child is standing upright. It should never be given to babies under 12 months, to a child who is crying or to a child who has difficulty swallowing.

Due to its oily texture, children often find mineral oil unpleasant to swallow on its own. Mixing it with orange juice, flavored milk, yogurt or ice cream helps to disguise the oily taste. Putting it in the freezer to make it ice cold also helps.

If you see an oily film on the water after your child has had a bowel movement, this means the dose is too high. The dose should be lowered until the film disappears.

There have been concerns that mineral oil may interfere with the absorption of some vitamins. However, there appears to be no clear evidence for this.[28,29]

3. Lactulose

Lactulose is an osmotic laxative which draws water into the lower bowel making stools soft and easy to pass. Compared to PEG, lactulose is extremely mild. Lactulose is a very popular choice for treating constipation in children and is known to be very gentle and safe for long term use. *However,* for a child who has been withholding for many months or years, lactulose is usually far too mild to be of benefit, even at high doses.

Before my son was prescribed PEG, he took lactulose for six months in ever increasing doses. This was on the advice of my doctor who thought initially, as I did, that we were dealing with straightforward constipation. Unfortunately, lactulose had no effect at all on his withholding. In fact, his bowel movements became even less frequent during the time he was taking it.

Lactulose can, however, be effective if your child has been stool withholding for less than a couple of months. It can also be effective for babies who are withholding.

Lactulose comes as a sweet-tasting liquid which children usually find easy to take. It can be given on its own, or mixed with water or juice. It usually takes 48 hours to have an effect. Common side effects include gas, bloating and abdominal cramps. Lactulose is not suitable for children who are lactose intolerant.

When to Come off Laxatives

I cannot stress enough the importance of *not* stopping your child's medication too soon. It can take many months, even years, to conquer a withholding habit. Remember, the length of time that your child has been withholding is usually the length of time it takes them to stop withholding once the right course of treatment is started.

Successful treatment often involves keeping your child on laxatives for quite a bit longer than you might think necessary *and* at a higher dose than you might feel comfortable with. It's tempting to stop the medication as soon as your child starts going regularly. However, stopping too soon often results in a return to infrequent bowel movements. Just because your child starts going regularly doesn't mean that they're not still trying their very hardest to hold on.

As a rough guideline, once your child has been having at least five complete bowel movements per week for three months, without any fear or resistance, this is a good time to try reducing the dose. Laxatives should be tapered slowly over several months rather than weeks. If the number of bowel movements per week decreases, quickly return to the previous dose for a further month before trying to cut down again.[3]

In the long term, we're aiming for at least one complete bowel movement per day. Some children will achieve once-a-day quite quickly while others will take longer. If the rectum has become very enlarged it probably needs to shrink back to its normal size before bowel movements can become frequent again. As we've seen, my son only achieved once-a-day some months *after* coming off laxatives.

Have Regular Follow-Ups with a Healthcare Professional

Your child should be monitored closely by a doctor, or other healthcare provider, during the disimpaction stage of treatment. Then, regular follow-up visits are recommended during the maintenance phase (about once a month). It's also important to continue with follow-ups once your child comes off laxatives (about every three to four months).

Stay *Very* Vigilant[3] After Your Child Comes off Laxatives

Once your child is off laxatives altogether, you need to monitor them closely for signs of constipation and infrequent bowel movements for *at least* a year afterwards, preferably longer if your child has had a long term issue. You also need to pay close attention to their diet and continue with the daily "toilet sit". (See Chapter 6 for more on diet and the daily toilet sit).

Dealing With Relapses - Don't Throw the Laxatives Away too Soon!

It's not uncommon for children to slide back into stool withholding some time after coming off laxatives, just when you think you're home and dry. Relapses are common if laxatives are tapered too quickly or too soon.

The key to long term recovery is to monitor the frequency of your child's bowel movements very closely. Once off medication, if three or so days pass without a bowel movement, a short course of laxatives may be required or another disimpaction may be needed.

Sometimes parents assume that a relapse happens because the laxatives have made their child's bowels "lazy" or dependent. However, this is very unlikely. A relapse will almost certainly be due to the return of the withholding habit.

How Many Bowel Movements Per Day is Normal?

The frequency of children's bowel movements varies widely, and parents are often confused about what's normal once their child comes off laxatives. Once-a-day is a good guideline. However, for some children, three times a day will be normal while for others it will be every other day. What's *most* important is that bowel movements are easy and pain-free and that your child goes willingly and without fear or distress.

As a guideline, the average number of complete bowel movements per day in healthy children is roughly as follows:[30]

0-3 months (breast fed)	2.9
0-3 months (formula fed)	2.0
6-12 months	1.8
1-3 years	1.4
Over 3 years	1.0

Keep Stocked Up With Medication

Remember to keep stocked up, well in advance, with your chosen laxative and with any food or drink needed for mixing it with. Suddenly stopping your child's medication, even for a couple of days, can cause them to relapse straight back to their old ways.

If a prescription is needed for your child's medication, this may take several days to come through so you need to plan ahead. And if you're going on vacation, it's essential to continue with your child's medication while you're away. A week off could undo all the hard work you've put in so far.

CHAPTER 5: Key Points

- Laxatives play an essential role in the treatment of stool withholding and encopresis. With the right dose, they make it extremely difficult for your child to hold on. Experiencing easy, pain-free, bowel movements *many* times over slowly breaks the vicious cycle of pain and fear.

- A long course of daily laxative medication, often for *at least* six months or more, and at quite a high initial dose, is usually the recommended treatment if your child has been withholding for some time.

- If your child is impacted, it's essential to clear the impaction first with a high dose of laxatives *before* moving on to the lower maintenance dose. Soiling should resolve gradually as the rectum returns to its normal size and functioning. However, further impactions must be prevented or soiling is likely to return.

- Enemas and suppositories can be distressing for children and are not usually recommended unless oral laxatives have failed to bring results.

- Parents' fears about the safety of laxatives often lead them to give laxatives on-and-off, at too low a dose, or to taper the medication off too soon. This usually results in repeated relapses. Giving a dose sporadically, or that's too low, is usually as good as doing nothing at all and simply wastes precious time. Parents should rest assured that the safety profile of laxatives today is very good.

- Taking the recommended dose of laxative consistently each day, *without fail,* is usually the fastest route to resolving your child's withholding. They may end up taking *less* medication, in total, with this approach than with a stop-start approach over many years.

- Polyethylene Glycol 3350 (PEG) is one of the most effective laxatives for stool withholding. Common brand names are

MiraLAX in the United States and RestoraLAX and Lax-A-Day in Canada. PEG has few side effects and can be used safely, over long periods, with children of all ages including babies.

- If your child struggles with the volume of liquid that needs taking with PEG, the dose of PEG can be reduced and a stimulant laxative or stool softener added. *Or,* if your child has no success with PEG at all, stimulant laxatives are safe to use on their own, or with a stool softener or a lubricant laxative.

- Lactulose can be effective for babies who stool withhold, and for children who have been withholding for less than a couple of months. However, lactulose is usually *far too* mild for a child with a long term withholding problem.

- It's important *not* to stop your child's medication too soon. Once they've been having at least five complete bowel movements per week for about three months, then the dose can slowly be reduced. The long term goal is one bowel movement per day. This may take time if the rectum has become very enlarged and needs to return to its normal size.

- When your child comes off laxatives, you should continue to closely monitor the frequency of their bowel movements for at least a year afterwards and to watch for signs of constipation and withholding. The key to recovery is to keep your child as regular as possible, for as long as possible. Follow-up visits with a healthcare professional are recommended.

CHAPTER 6: What Else Can You Do To Help?

In this chapter, we'll look at some other very important things you can do to help your child. Using laxatives *in combination with* the strategies we'll be outlining is much more effective than using laxatives alone.

1. The Daily "Toilet Sit"

We mentioned the daily toilet sit in Chapter 3. However, I want to discuss it further because it's such an important routine to establish. If your child is already toilet trained, or in the process of toilet training, scheduling one daily toilet sit for pooping, at the *same* time *every* day, in either the morning or evening, can assist their recovery for several important reasons:

a)   scheduling either a morning or evening sit greatly reduces your child's need to go during the day while at school or preschool, where many children withhold because they dislike using the bathroom there. It's a good idea to establish this routine even if your child hasn't yet started school or preschool.

b)   the daily toilet sit creates an easy and predictable routine in your child's life. With practice, it should become an ingrained habit which they carry out on automatic pilot each day. Soon, it will become part of their natural bodily rhythm to go at the scheduled time.

c) the daily toilet sit makes it easier for you to monitor how often your child has a bowel movement. Without a strict routine, it's easy to lose track of when your child last used the bathroom and skipping bowel movements will delay progress.

For many families, evenings are more relaxed than mornings as there's no rush to leave the home. Going in the evening may also ensure a better night's sleep for your child by eliminating any urges to go during the night. Our bowels often become active after a meal, so early evening can be a natural time for children to go anyway. If you're an early riser, then a morning sit should work just as well, as long as your child isn't rushed or pressured.

For the over three's, one toilet sit per day for pooping is usually quite enough. Any more than this can cause them unnecessary stress. However, all children are different and some may need two daily toilet sits per day. Toilet trained children *under* three years usually benefit from a morning *and* evening sit.

The evening toilet sit certainly worked wonders with my son. From the age of three and a half, I would prompt him to sit on the toilet every night at about 6.30pm. This became part of his bedtime routine along with tooth-brushing and face-washing. He soon developed a natural bodily urge to go at this time and he continues with this routine, without thinking, several years on.

You should emphasize to your child that it doesn't matter if they're unable to poop during their toilet sit. You can still praise them for trying. The important thing is that they sit on the potty or toilet for at least 5-10 minutes *and* that they do some pushing while they're there - simply sitting is not enough. Offering rewards for their efforts can help to establish this routine.

A toy or a book can be a useful distraction while they sit. And, as we've already seen, giving them some privacy can be helpful for some children.

It may take a while to train your child to perform at your chosen time. Most of us have a bowel movement only when we get that unmistakable urge to go. In your child's case, we're trying to make them go at a set time when they may not have a strong urge. It's still possible, of course, to pass a stool without any urge at all. However, over time, your child should start to get a genuine urge at the time of their scheduled sit.

If you want to encourage things along, a warm bath beforehand can help. So, too, can a tummy massage, a hot drink, or a hot-water bottle placed on the abdomen. I heard of one parent getting their child to bounce on a trampoline to get things moving!

Prompting Your Child to Have Their Daily Toilet Sit

I continued to remind my son to have his evening toilet sit for nearly two years *after* he came off laxatives. This may seem like a long time; however, if you don't prompt, your child is likely to skip bowel movements and before you know it, the withholding habit has returned.

Young children are unlikely to brush their teeth or go to bed on time without prompting, so reminding them to have their poop each day isn't a major inconvenience. Hopefully, as they get used to the routine, they'll do it willingly.

Once your child comes off laxatives and has been having easy, regular bowel movements for about a year, you may want to stop prompting to see what happens. Holidays and weekends are a good time to try this.

Toilet Sitting Position

Toilet sitting position is surprisingly important when it comes to stool withholding. Before the invention of the modern day toilet, humans used to squat on the ground to poop. Our intestine has a natural kink in it just before the rectum. The squatting position, with the knees up near the chest, forces the muscle around the rectum to relax and makes the kink straighten out. This allows stools to pass out easily and with little effort.

It's therefore much more difficult for your child to hold on if their knees are raised up while they sit on the toilet. This can be achieved by resting their feet on a box or step, so that their knees are higher than their waist. It also helps if they lean forward slightly with their elbows resting on their knees. A toilet seat insert is usually needed until the age of about five to make the seat smaller and more comfortable. Most potties enable a sitting position quite close to squatting so it's not necessary to raise the feet.

2. Rewards

Offering a reward for a successful bowel movement can be a *huge* incentive for many children and played a major role in my son's recovery. It always amazed me that the promise of just one square of chocolate would have him sitting on the toilet in an instant, where minutes before he'd been screaming and protesting.

While I don't think rewarding your child with candy is ever a habit to be encouraged, if it leads to a successful bowel movement it's a valuable tool, as long as you stick to small quantities. Limiting candy *just* for rewards can give it extra power.

Of course, not all children will be impressed with sugar. You may have to offer other incentives such as a small toy, money for the piggy bank, stickers, a magazine or a favorite TV program or DVD. Being allowed the use of an iPad, or similar gadget, can be a big incentive for older children.

Make Rewards Visible

Making the reward visible to your child *before* they produce the desired result can make all the difference. Some parents achieve success by taping the reward in a clear plastic bag, high up on the bathroom wall, so that their child can see it while they sit.

Initially, if your child's resistance is extreme, you may need to offer a reward just to get them to enter the bathroom. Another reward can then be offered for sitting on the toilet and then another for a successful bowel movement - one piece of candy for each step, for example. Later, when these steps have been mastered, you can limit rewards to a successful bowel movement.

Small rewards are of course best, as this is going to be a regular outlay. As your child starts to recover, longer term rewards may work better - a more expensive toy or a trip to the movies, for five poops in a week, for example. Then slowly, over time, you can tail off the rewards without your child noticing.

Praising your child for their successes on the toilet is to be encouraged but don't go too over the top. We don't want them to feel that your reason to live depends on them having a bowel movement!

3. Buy a Year Chart

Your family doctor or pediatrician may advise you to keep a detailed daily log recording each dose of laxative and the time and consistency of each bowel movement. While I've no doubt this is a very good idea, sticking to this type of diary can be stressful and time consuming, particularly for long periods. I certainly found it a bit of a chore.

What I found to be much easier and more effective was to use a large calendar or "planner" for the whole year. This is the type you can stick on the wall which shows each month running horizontally across the page. These can be bought very cheaply in stores or on the internet. I highly recommend any parent with a stool withholding child to purchase one.

All you need to do is place a tick or sticker on the relevant day of your chart whenever your child has a poop. Your child may enjoy being involved in this too, but primarily this is for *your* benefit.

This type of chart makes it easy to see when your child last had a bowel movement and gives you a clear picture of how things are progressing over the year. It also helps you to spot a relapse easily and to judge when to start tapering off laxatives.

Over time, you should see the number of bowel movements per month gradually increase - a pattern you might not notice so easily with a detailed weekly log. It's a good idea to continue with your year chart for up to a year *after* your child comes off laxatives.

Eventually, you'll be putting a tick or sticker on every single day of your chart and that's when you know your child is well on the road to recovery.

4. Create a Simple Routine and Stick to It

It helps enormously if you can create a simple and easy routine for your child that you can repeat each day, at the *same* time, with very little thought or effort. You may need to carry out this routine for many months or more. If it's easy, you're much more likely to stick to it for the long term.

The quickest route to your child's recovery is to carry out your routine with military precision each day, without fail. Skipping a day here and there will delay progress. Great discipline and patience is required here, but your efforts *will* pay off.

I had a simple daily drill for my son which went as follows:

1. **Breakfast time:** MiraLAX dissolved in orange juice
2. **Dinner time:** MiraLAX dissolved in orange juice
3. **Bed time:** Toilet sit with reward for bowel movement; Update year chart as necessary.

I followed this formula religiously, each day, for six months. It quickly became completely automatic for us both. I just had to remember to keep stocked up with medication, orange juice and rewards. I continued with the daily toilet sit and the year chart long after my son came off laxatives.

5. Keep Constipation at Bay

Constipation is the most common trigger for stool withholding so we want to avoid constipation at all costs, particularly once your child comes off laxatives. Even a mild bout of constipation could cause them to start withholding again.

Keeping a close eye on your child's diet is the best way to avoid constipation. It's a good idea to start working on their diet while they're taking laxatives so that when they *stop* taking them, good eating habits are already well established.

Foods Which Can *Prevent* Constipation

Foods which help to prevent constipation include:

- Brown whole-wheat bread
- Brown whole-wheat pasta
- Brown rice
- Oatmeal or other high-fiber cereals such as Shredded Wheat, All-Bran, Bran Flakes, Grape-Nuts or granola
- Baked potatoes (with skin)
- Sweet potatoes
- Beans including baked beans and chick peas
- Fruit especially oranges, pears, peaches, kiwis and mangoes
- Dried fruits such as prunes, apricots, figs, raisins or dates
- Prune juice and pear juice
- Vegetables especially broccoli, carrots, peas and corn
- Avocados
- Popcorn (plain)
- Lentils
- Nuts (not suitable for children under five due to choking risk)
- Peanut butter, particularly the crunchy variety.

Switching from white to *brown* bread, pasta and rice is a good step to take. Mixing brown pasta with white pasta can help your child adjust to the taste.

If your child is a fussy-eater and you have difficulty getting them to eat high-fiber foods, there are various fiber supplements, such as psyllium husks or glucomannan, which can be added to food or juice. Fiber supplements are not particularly effective when it comes to stool withholding. However, they *can* help with occasional constipation once your child has overcome their withholding. Fiber supplements should be introduced gradually to avoid gas, bloating and cramps.

Foods Which Can *Cause* Constipation

The following foods can contribute to constipation and should be reduced or avoided:

- Fast-foods, processed foods or high fat foods such as pizzas, burgers and packaged/frozen meals - these are usually all low in fiber.
- High sugar foods such as cookies, pastries and cakes - again, these tend to be low in fiber.
- Bananas
- Dairy products such as milk, cheese and yogurt. As we discussed in Chapter 3, dairy products should *not* be eliminated but reduced to 2-3 small servings per day (see page 27).

Keep Active

Keeping active is another good way to stimulate the gut and to keep food moving along the intestine. If your child spends a lot of time sitting or lying down, it's a good idea to switch off the TV and get them to take some exercise. At least one hour per day of activity is to be encouraged.

Drink Plenty of Fluids

We know that dehydration can contribute to constipation by making stools hard and more difficult to pass.[31] If your child's urine is dark yellow in color, it's a sign that they should be drinking more.

It's helpful to offer drinks, preferably water, to your child regularly through the day, particularly with meals, and to keep a water bottle close at hand. Drinking plenty of fluids is particularly important if your child is taking laxatives.

Many schools now encourage children to take a water bottle into class. If this isn't the policy at your child's school or preschool, it's worth asking if this is allowed.

As a guideline, the daily fluid intake for children, in the form of drinks, should be roughly as follows:[32]

1-2 year olds	3½ - 4½ glasses
2-3 year olds	4½ - 5 glasses
4-8 year olds	5½ - 6½ glasses
9-13 year olds (girls)	6½ - 7½ glasses
9-13 year olds (boys)	7½ - 8½ glasses
14-18 year olds (girls)	7 - 9 glasses
14-18 year olds (boys)	9 - 12 glasses

1 glass = 7fl oz (200mls) of water or any other drink.

The amount of fluid your child needs will, of course, increase in hot weather and with physical activity.

Tackle Constipation Immediately

It's important to watch closely for constipation once your child has come off laxatives and appears to have overcome their withholding. Constipation needs to be tackled straight away in a child with a history of stool withholding to avoid a relapse. If your child strains while on the toilet and their stools are solid, hard and dark in color, or look like small pellets, this indicates constipation. A short course of laxatives may be needed, together with some changes to their diet.

6. Back Off and Change the Subject!

Parents of a stool withholding child often reach a point where they barely talk to their child about anything other than the subject of pooping. Sometimes the whole family becomes engrossed with the issue too.

This is a very common and easy trap to fall into and I was definitely guilty of this with my son. I would constantly ask him if he needed a poop, endlessly harass him to sit on the toilet and then desperately urge him to push. I'm sure he was very aware of my feelings of intense frustration and disappointment when he failed to produce a result.

I would also have sessions where I'd try to persuade him to stop holding on. Of course, this was all a complete waste of time and effort. It simply created an extremely tense and unhappy home environment and put an immense pressure on my son's small shoulders.

If you've fallen into this trap, the best advice I can give is to back off and change the subject when you're with your child, as much as you humanly can. No amount of talking, cajoling, fussing or pressuring is going to stop them withholding. In fact, it's probably going to make things worse.

Try to change the subject completely, focus on other things and adopt a relaxed and nonchalant manner in front of your child in relation to their toileting. When you do this, you'll probably notice a huge amount of tension disappearing from them and everyone else involved.

7. Explain About Poop and the Body

Once you've had a good break from talking to your child about their withholding, it *can* help to have a few relaxed chats with them about poop and the body. I suspect a lot of 2-3 year olds believe that if they hold on to their poop for long enough it will simply disappear.

It's helpful to explain to them about the journey that food takes as it passes through their body from their mouth, to their stomach and along their intestine. You can say that on its journey, the good parts of the food are taken out and what's left over is turned into poop. You can stress that poop *has* to come out of their body, one way or another, and that holding on will *never* make it go away.

When my son grasped this, some of his resistance definitely fell away. At the age of three, he was certainly very interested to learn about how his body worked.

It's also a good idea to let your child talk freely about poop in a relaxed and open way and to teach them that it's not a disgusting, shameful or naughty subject. We all have to poop, after all.

There are some excellent illustrated books available for young children which can help you with this topic. I recommend the following:

-   *"Everyone Poops"* by Taro Gomi;

-   *"It Hurts When I Poop! A Story For Children Who Are Scared To Use The Potty"* by Howard J. Bennett;

-   *"I Can't, I Won't, No Way!: A Book For Children Who Refuse To Poop"* by Tracey Vessillo.

Older, school-age, children may benefit from learning about stool withholding in a bit more detail. You can explain what may have triggered their stool withholding and why they need to take laxatives. If they have a soiling issue, you should stress that it's not their fault, but due to soft poop seeping out around a hard impacted lump. The more they understand, the more relaxed and optimistic they will feel about the whole issue.

8. The Role of Teddy

A favorite teddy bear or stuffed animal can play a useful role with younger children. My son took great comfort from pretending that his teddy was also a stool withholder. They would both sit side by side on separate potties in the bathroom. Teddy also had to take laxatives which encouraged my son to take his own medication.

Children have wonderful imaginations and you can take advantage of this in any way that helps - the more creative you can be the better. I came across one mother who achieved results after sprinkling "fairy dust" over the toilet and telling her daughter it would magically make her poop come out.

9. Talk to Staff at Your Child's School, Preschool or Day Care Center

It can be particularly stressful if your child's stool withholding coincides with the start of school, preschool or day care. It's a very good idea to talk to a teacher, or other member of staff, about your child's withholding so that the issue can be dealt with sensitively and in the right way, should the need arise. This is particularly important if your child is on a high dose of laxatives or has a soiling problem.

Building a supportive relationship with a member of staff who is knowledgeable about stool withholding can be immensely helpful. Some teachers may have encountered this issue before so don't be afraid or embarrassed to talk to them. Lend them a copy of this book if necessary. If there's a school nurse or school counselor, it can be extremely helpful to get them on your side too.

There are a few issues you may need to discuss with staff at your child's school, preschool or day care center:

i)   If your child has a soiling problem, find out if any staff are able to deal with this. Schools often have a policy about how they will deal with a soiling incident.

It's usually outside a teacher's job description to clean up a child and deal with soiled underwear. Parents may be called to the school to change their child and collect dirty clothing. However, at some schools there may be staff who are prepared to deal with this. Your child will obviously need to take spare clothing to school for any soiling accidents.

ii) Staff should be made aware that your child has no control over this type of soiling and should *never* be scolded or punished for it.

iii) If soiling is an issue, your child will almost certainly be impacted. A high dose of laxatives will be needed to clear the impaction. The disimpaction phase can be messy so you may need to take your child out of school for a few days to deal with it at home. Teachers need to understand the importance of clearing an impaction as quickly as possible and that time off school may be necessary.

iv) Some children may benefit from access to a private bathroom at school or preschool. It's worth checking with teachers if this is possible. Stress to staff the importance of giving your child privacy while they poop and that this can be helpful for their recovery.

v) Where possible, staff should allow your child to use the bathroom whenever they need to, rather than restrict them to specific times.

vi) Preschools often have a policy about the age at which children are expected to be out of diapers. If your child needs to wear diapers longer than usual, hopefully staff will show some flexibility if they understand that stool withholding often delays toilet training.

vii) Some stool withholding children may still be in diapers or training pants when they start school. This may be because they're on a high dose of laxatives or because their toilet training has been delayed due to their withholding. Again, it helps if teachers have a good understanding of stool withholding and the difficult issues you are dealing with. You can stress that you are taking the appropriate steps to tackle the problem as quickly as possible.

viii) For a toilet trained child at preschool or in day care who will only poop in a diaper but not in the potty or toilet, staff need to understand the importance of allowing your child to use a diaper, just for pooping, until bowel movements become easy and regular. This step can greatly assist your child.

ix) Staff should understand that any irritable or difficult behavior on your child's part may well be due to their stool withholding and that your child needs to be treated sensitively and with great understanding.

Staff should also be aware that your child may go through phases of extreme discomfort and distress when they're trying to hold on. They may need to be gently encouraged, but not forced, to visit the bathroom.

x) If your child needs to take a dose of laxative medication during the day, staff obviously need to be informed so that they can help with this.

xi) It's helpful if staff ensure that water is available for your child at all times - taking a water bottle is a good idea. Drinking plenty of fluids helps prevent constipation and is also important if your child is on laxatives.

10. Talk to Anyone Else Involved in the Care of Your Child

If anyone else takes care of your child on a regular basis such as relatives, friends, nannies or au pairs, you should let them know about your child's situation. This is particularly important if your child ever stays away from home. Overlooking important details like the daily toilet sit, medication, rewards, privacy and not punishing your child for withholding or soiling, could delay progress or cause a relapse.

11. Seek a Second Opinion if Necessary

If any healthcare provider tells you that your child will simply "grow out" of their stool withholding, or that a change of diet is all that's needed, they're clearly not up-to-speed on the subject. If this is your experience, I would strongly urge you to seek a second opinion elsewhere.

Fortunately, there *are* doctors and other healthcare professionals who are knowledgeable about stool withholding. However, I know of many parents, worldwide, who have struggled to find the right help and I certainly experienced difficulties with this myself. Having the support of a professional who fully understands this subject can make all the difference to your child's recovery.

CHAPTER 6: Key Points

- For toilet trained children, enforcing a daily "toilet sit" at the *same* time *every* day can greatly assist their recovery. An evening (or morning) toilet sit reduces the need for a bowel movement while at school or preschool, where children often withhold because they dislike using the bathroom there.

- Using a box or step to raise your child's feet while they sit on the toilet allows the intestine to "unkink" and the muscle around the rectum to relax. This helps stools to pass out more easily and makes it much more difficult for your child to hold on.

- Offering small rewards to your child for each bowel movement can play a major part in breaking the withholding habit. Rewards are particularly effective if you make them visible to your child *before* they use the bathroom.

- Buying a year chart or "planner" and placing a tick or sticker on each day that your child has a bowel movement, is a simple and effective way to monitor progress. It allows you to spot a relapse easily and to see a clear pattern of improvement over the year.

- Creating a simple daily routine around your child's medication and toileting means you're more likely to stick to it for the long term. Giving medication at the same time each day, enforcing the toilet sit with rewards as necessary, and updating your year chart is usually all that's needed on a daily basis.

- It's essential to avoid constipation by monitoring your child's diet, particularly once they've come off laxatives. If your child does become constipated this needs to be tackled immediately to prevent a relapse.

- Pressuring your child to use the toilet and endlessly focusing on their withholding puts them under great stress. It's best to avoid the subject, as much as possible, and adopt a relaxed and nonchalant attitude to their toileting.

- Very young children often think that holding on to their poop will make it disappear. It helps to explain how food passes through their body, turns into poop and then *has* to come out. Older children may benefit from learning about stool withholding in more detail.

- For children at school, preschool or in day care, it's important to discuss their withholding with a teacher, or other staff member, so it can be handled sensitively and appropriately. It may help to involve the school nurse or counselor, if there is one. Anyone else who cares for your child on a regular basis should also be made aware of the withholding issue, particularly if your child ever stays away from home.

- If you have any difficulty obtaining the right help and advice from your child's doctor, or other healthcare provider, seek a second opinion. Stool withholding is still a widely misunderstood problem and it's important that your child receives appropriate support.

CHAPTER 7: A Final Word

I came across some very sad stories during the course of writing this book. There are clearly many children, worldwide, who are currently battling with a long term soiling and withholding problem. Some appear to be receiving either the wrong type of help, or no help at all. Often, the problem isn't detected early on, and children are frequently being treated with doses of laxative which are too low to have any effect.

Left untreated, stool withholding can bring untold misery to children and their families. It's heart breaking to hear of children being bullied and ostracized at school because of a chronic soiling issue. However, many of these stories could be prevented.

You'll have gathered by now that a head-on, military-style, approach to treatment, often involving high doses of laxatives for many months or longer, is what usually brings results. Sometimes parents see this method as rather aggressive and will shun laxatives in favor of a "natural" approach involving diet. This *may* work if the problem is caught very early on, but often the "natural" approach simply wastes precious time.

Cast Aside Your Fears About Laxatives

In an ideal world, we'd all opt for a natural approach without resorting to medication. However, stool withholding is not the same as straightforward constipation. A fairly "aggressive" approach is often needed, particularly for longer term withholders. The alternative is to drag this issue out for years and possibly into early teens or beyond. I would urge parents to cast aside their fears about medication. With the right dose, laxatives are very safe and very effective.

The Magic Formula

Laxatives are most effective when they're used in combination with the various strategies and tactics we've discussed throughout this book. What's also required is a great deal of sensitivity and compassion in dealing with your child, *and* you must stick religiously to your daily routine and follow treatment right through to the very end. This, I believe, is the magic formula.

Recovery Takes Time

Recovery is about retraining your child's bowel *and* brain. Like learning to drive a car or play the piano, it takes time to learn a new skill. Daily repetition over many months, and sometimes years, is needed for the new habit to completely take hold. However, your patience and persistence *will* be rewarded.

Can We Prevent Stool Withholding?

We know that constipation is the most common trigger for stool withholding. The key to prevention is clearly to avoid constipation, or to catch it at its very earliest stage. I believe this could prevent many, if not most, cases of stool withholding. Constipation in children should, therefore, be taken very seriously.

Parents don't seem to be as tuned into constipation as they used to be. My parents were born in the 1930's and they both recall the great emphasis in those days on keeping children "regular". It was commonplace back then for children to be dosed frequently with old-fashioned remedies like syrup of figs and castor oil.

For some reason, this emphasis on preventing constipation seems to have fallen out of fashion. I would love to see this change. I'd also like to see the day when most parents have heard of stool withholding and can talk about it freely and openly without having to suffer in silence.

Education & Awareness

Parents clearly need to be made more aware of this subject. I am certain that I could have prevented my son's stool withholding had I been aware of the following facts:

- painful constipation sometimes causes children to stool withhold, so preventing constipation is very important;
- constipation should be tackled as quickly and as early as possible in children if it does arise;
- drinking too much cow's milk can lead to constipation;
- rushed or pressured toilet training can cause children to stool withhold;
- children in diapers who hide before having a bowel movement are often constipated and more likely to start withholding;
- children who refuse the potty/toilet and will only go in a diaper are often constipated and more likely to start withholding.

However, it's not just parents who need this information. Stool withholding is still widely misunderstood even amongst healthcare professionals. I believe *anyone* involved in the care of children should have a basic understanding of this subject. I am sure that a widespread increase in awareness would significantly reduce the incidence of stool withholding and spare many families across the world a great deal of misery.

The Joy of Recovery

There's no joy like it when your child starts to have regular bowel movements again. As my son recovered, not only did his mood and behavior transform, but there were other unexpected improvements: his appetite returned, he gained weight, his bloated abdomen disappeared and he started sleeping soundly through the night for the first time. Great joy and relief was felt throughout the family. I hope this book will help you to achieve the same happy outcome.

Your Feedback

I want the information given here to be as useful and up-to-date as possible. If you have any feedback, I would be very grateful to hear from you. You can contact me at www.stoolwithholding.com.

USEFUL WEBSITES & INTERNET FORUMS

www.theinsandoutsofpoop.com

This is Dr Thomas DuHamel's website, author of "The Ins and Outs of Poop". Here you'll find a wealth of information about constipation and withholding. You can also email "Dr Tom" with your queries.

www.ucanpooptoo.com

This website offers an online program for overcoming encopresis. It also contains lots of useful articles and information about how to deal with encopresis and withholding.

Internet forums where you can talk to other parents about your child's issues:

www.circleofmoms.com
www.cafemom.com
www.mothering.com

REFERENCES

1. Taubman, B. (1997) Toilet Training and Toileting Refusal for Stool Only: A Prospective Study. *Pediatrics*, 99, 54-58.

2. Cohn, Anthony. (2007) *Constipation, Withholding and Your Child: A Family Guide to Soiling and Wetting.* London: Jessica Kingsley Publishers.

3. DuHamel, Thomas R. (2012) *The Ins and Outs of Poop: A Guide to Treating Childhood Constipation.* Seattle: Maret Publishing.

4. Cohn, A. (2005) Stool Withholding Presenting as a Cause of Non-Epileptic Seizures. *Developmental Medicine & Child Neurology*, 47, 703-705.

5. Gidding, S., Dennison, B., Birch, L., Daniels, S., Gilman, M., Lichtenstein, A. et al (2006) American Academy of Pediatrics: Dietary Recommendations for Children and Adolescents: A Guide for Practitioners. *Pediatrics*, 117(2), 544-559.

6. United States Department of Agriculture "What Counts as a Cup in the Dairy Group?", www.choosemyplate.gov

7. Iacono, G., Cavataio, F., Montalto, G., Florena, A., Tumminello, M., Soresi M. et al (1998) Intolerance of Cow's Milk and Chronic Constipation in Children. *The New England Journal of Medicine*, 339(16), 1100-1104.

8. Blum, N., Taubman, B. & Nemeth, N. (2004) During Toilet Training, Constipation Occurs Before Stool Toileting Refusal. *Pediatrics*, 113(6), e520-522.

9. Taubman, B., Blum, N. & Nemeth, N. (2003) Children Who Hide While Defecating Before They Have Completed Toilet Training: A Prospective Study. *Archives of Pediatrics & Adolescent Medicine*, 157(12), 1190-1192.

10. Taubman, B., Blum, N. & Nemeth, N. (2003) Stool Toileting Refusal: A Prospective Intervention Targeting Parental Behaviour. *Archives of Pediatrics & Adolescent Medicine*, 157(12), 1193-1196.

11. Lundblad, B. & Hellström, A. (2005) Perceptions of School Toilets as a Cause for Irregular Toilet Habits Among School Children Aged 6 to 16 years. *Journal of School Health*, 75(4), 125-128.

12. Vernon, S., Lundblad, B. & Hellström, A. (2003) Children's Experiences of School Toilets Present a Risk to Their Physical and Psychological Health. *Child: Care, Health & Development*, 29(1), 47-53.

13. Blum, N., Taubman, B. & Osborne, M. (1997) Behavioral Characteristics of Children With Stool Toileting Refusal. *Pediatrics*, 99(1), 50-53.

14. Friman, P., Mathews, J., Finney, J., Christophersen, E. & Leibowitz, J. (1988) Do Encopretic Children Have Clinically Significant Behaviour Problems? *Pediatrics*, 82, 407-409.

15. Brooks, R., Copen, R., Cox, D., Morris, J., Borowitz, S. & Sutphen, J. (2000) Review of the Treatment Literature for Encopresis, Functional Constipation, and Stool-Toileting Refusal. *Annals of Behavioral Medicine*, 22(3), 260-267.

16. McElhanon, B., McCracken, C., Karpen, S. & Sharp, W. (2014) Gastrointestinal Symptoms in Autism Spectrum Disorder: A Meta-analysis. *Pediatrics*, 133(5), 872-883.

17. Constipation in Children and Young People: Diagnosis and Management of Idiopathic Childhood Constipation in Primary and Secondary Care (2010) *National Institute for Health and Care Excellence (NICE)*, Clinical Guideline 99.

18. Wald, A. (2003) Is Chronic Use of Stimulant Laxatives Harmful to the Colon? *Journal of Clinical Gastroenterology*, 36(5), 386-389.

19. McClung, H. & Potter, C. (2004) Rational Use of Laxatives in Children. *Advances In Pediatrics*, 51:231-62.

20. Müller-Lissner, S., Kamm, M., Scarpignato, C. & Wald, A. (2005) Myths and Misconceptions About Chronic Constipation. *American Journal of Gastroenterology*, 100(1), 232-242.

21. DiPalma, J., DeRidder, P., Orlando, R., Kolts, B. & Cleveland, M. (2000) A Randomized, Placebo-Controlled, Multicenter Study of the Safety and Efficacy of a New Polyethylene Glycol Laxative. *American Journal of Gastroenterology*, 95(2), 446–450.

22. Candy, D., Edwards, D. & Geraint, M. (2006) Treatment of Faecal Impaction With Polyethelene Glycol Plus Electrolytes (PGE + E) Followed by a Double-blind Comparison of PEG + E Versus Lactulose as Maintenance Therapy. *Journal of Pediatric Gastroenterology & Nutrition*, 43(1), 65-70.

23. Bharucha, A., Dorn, S., Lembo, A. & Pressman, A. (2013) American Gastroenterological Association Medical Position Statement on Constipation. *Gastroenterology*, 144, 211-217.

24. Pashankar, D., Loening-Baucke, V. & Bishop, W. (2003) Safety of Polyethylene Glycol 3350 for the Treatment of Chronic Constipation in Children. *Archives of Pediatrics & Adolescent Medicine*, 157(7), 661-664.

25. Pashankar, D., Bishop, W. & Loening-Baucke, V. (2003) Long-term Efficacy of Polyethylene Glycol 3350 for the Treatment of Chronic Constipation in Children With and Without Encopresis. *Clinical Pediatrics*, 42(9), 815-819.

26. Loening-Baucke, V., Krishna, R. & Pashankar, D. (2004) Polyethylene Glycol 3350 Without Electrolytes for the Treatment of Functional Constipation in Infants and Toddlers. *Journal of Pediatric Gastroenterology and Nutrition*, 39(5), 536-539.

27. Michail, S., Gendy, E., Preud'Homme, D. & Mezoff, A. (2004) Polyethylene Glycol for Constipation in Children Younger Than Eighteen Months Old. *Journal of Pediatric Gastroenterology and Nutrition*, 39(2), 197-199.

28. Gal-Ezer, S. & Shaoul, R. (2006) The Safety of Mineral Oil in the Treatment of Constipation - A Lesson From Prolonged Overdose. *Clinical Pediatrics*, 45(9), 856-858.

29. Sharif, F., Crushell, E., O'Driscoll, K. & Bourke, B. (2001) Liquid Paraffin: A Reappraisal of its Role in the Treatment of Constipation. *Archives of Disease in Childhood*, 85, 121-124.

30. Fontana, M., Bianchi, C., Cataldo, F., Conti Nibali, S., Cucchiari, S., Gobio Casali, L. et al. (1989) Bowel Frequency in Healthy Children. *Acta Paediatrica Scandinavica*, 78, 682-684.

31. Arnaud, M. (2003) Mild Dehydration: A Risk Factor of Constipation? *European Journal of Clinical Nutrition*, 57(2), S88-95.

32. European Food Safety Authority. Scientific Opinion on Dietary Reference Values for Water. (2010) *EFSA Journal*, 8(3), 1459.

45546083R00054

Made in the USA
San Bernardino, CA
11 February 2017